THE CHILDBIRTH PICTURE BOOK

Table of contents

Pictures

Original text by Fran P. Hosken

Drawings by Marcia L. Williams

14th EDITION: Updated for 2016, with a tribute to Fran Hosken

Published by: Hesperian Health Guides

Hesperian Health Guides
2860 Telegraph Avenue, Oakland, California 94609 USA
www.hesperian.org

ISBN 978-1-942919-23-0

THE CHILDBIRTH PICTURE BOOK

A tribute to Fran Hosken

Fran Hosken wrote the first *Childbirth Picture Book,* illustrated by Marcia Williams, in 1981. She sent out nearly 100,000 copies from her home in Lexington, Massachusetts, USA. She gave publication rights to dozens of organizations around the world who translated the book into local languages and distributed many thousands more copies. Fran also founded the Women's International Network through which she edited and published over 100 quarterly issues of *Women's International Network News.* She published numerous articles and books on women's issues, the best known of which was the "Hosken Report on Female Genital Mutilation." She devised and promoted participatory programs to combat FGM and other practices destructive to women's health. She testified on women's issues before US Congressional Committees and spoke at major women's conferences.

Fran died in February, 2006 at the age of 86. The impact of her life is summarized in a moving tribute from Kpakiwa Aiah, from Sierra Leone, who had known and worked with Fran since 1985:

"The death has left a big pain and gap in the heart and minds of thousands if not millions of those who benefited directly or indirectly from The Childbirth Picture Book. *She will be remembered for her great work... To see a woman of substance sacrifice her time, energy, and resources to assist the least privileged depart in death is painful. That reminds me that whatever one decides to do must be done in good faith for which you will be remembered after you have passed away... What a great woman she has proved to be. When I return to the project site, both the project members and the entire community will observe 7 days of mourning for Fran Hosken. At the end of the 7 days, we shall conduct a memorial service for her at the UMC Church in Kono. Fran has been the brain and moral support behind our organization. May God grant her eternal rest."*

Women's reproductive health is still an issue

In 2016, Hesperian Health Guides took the baton passed by Fran's son, John Hosken, and Anne Merewood, Director of The Breastfeeding Center, to become responsible for the publication and distribution of *The Childbirth Picture Book.* We are grateful for the trust they have placed in us, especially since we remember and were inspired by Fran Hosken. We share Fran's insistence that the medical community recognize the importance of women's health issues and deal with them with respect, equality, and urgency. Central to achieving that is the empowerment of women and men with accurate information to dispel centuries of myths and misinformation about pregnancy, birth, and how women's bodies work. Unfortunately, the refusal to recognize a woman's right to understand and control her body continues to characterize both the medical and political systems in the US and throughout the world. Hesperian's commitment to producing and distributing *The Childbirth Picture Book* in English, Spanish, French, Arabic, Swahili, Somali, and hopefully additional languages, is part of the effort to help everyone everywhere take charge of their health.

Sarah Shannon, Executive Director
Hesperian Health Guides

THE CHILDBIRTH PICTURE BOOK

Introduction

This Picture Book presents the biological facts of reproduction shared by women all over the world, no matter what the country or society. Women everywhere experience the same joys and tribulations of childbearing, and the same health concerns. Regardless of where or how we live, we are conceived and born in the same way.

This book exists to make the human story of how we are made available to the largest number of people all over the world, regardless of language and literacy. Without reproduction, none of us would exist; therefore, the information on how we are made is essential to all of us. The story of this wonderful process is shown here in drawings, accompanied by short, factual explanations: it is presented from a woman's view. But, it is also addressed to men: because it is especially important that men — husbands/partners, fathers, and sons — begin to see the process of conception and birth from a woman's view, to understand how a child is created and what a woman goes through to give life.

Men have been kept away from childbirth in most societies. This book has been developed in the belief that since the creation of a child is a shared experience between a woman and a man, so should be its birth. This information should be shared, as the responsibilities and pleasures of children are shared.

The first need for women and men is to understand the marvelous process of nature that shapes the female body, so we can conceive and nurture a child. If you choose to have a baby, you also assume the responsibility to take good care of yourself. The role of the father-to-be is to support his partner throughout the process of creating life, to assure that she and the baby she carries are healthy and well cared for. To fulfill his responsibility in the creation of a healthy and happy family, he needs to know about childbirth and to understand this experience from a woman's view.

The failure to learn about the natural biological process of giving life, or how a baby is made, continues to be the cause of great suffering, pain and tragedy; quite needlessly. Millions of women and girls continue to live in fear and ignorance of their own bodies and life-giving functions. In many areas of the world, more women still die of childbirth than of any disease; yet this is entirely and easily preventable. The biological facts of reproduction continue to be the best kept secrets in many parts of the world, often distorted by damaging myths, taboos, and fears that threaten and debase the lives and dignity of women.

We hope that this book and program will be helpful by making the vital information on reproductive health accessible and available all over the world: it is designed for those who, so far, have not been reached with this vital information.

Fran Hosken

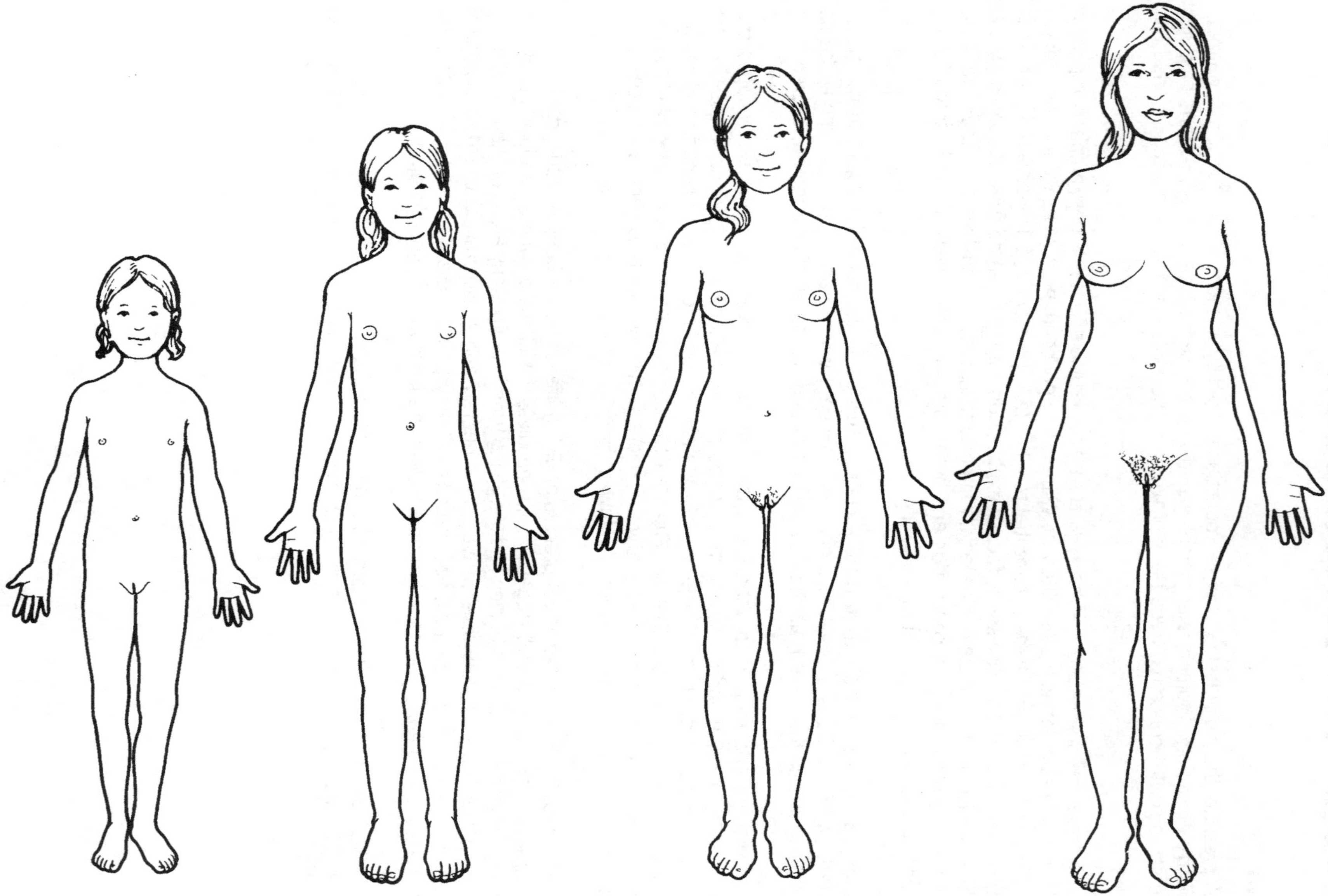

1. The female body: Growing from child to woman
Growing up to become a healthy woman takes many years: we need to wait until our bodies are big and strong enough to start childbearing.

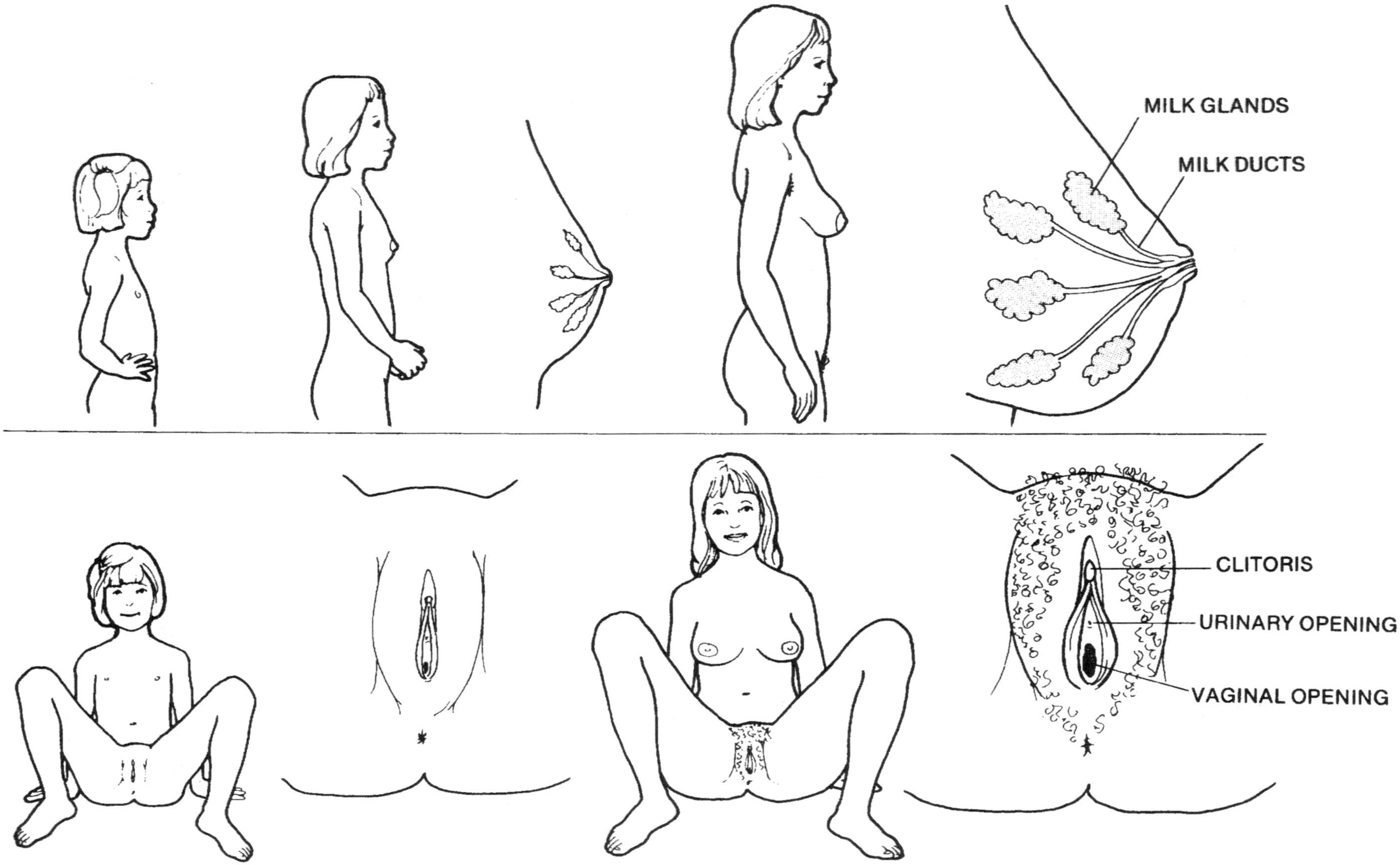

2. How the female body changes: the breasts and the genital organs
Changes of the female body take place both outside and inside.

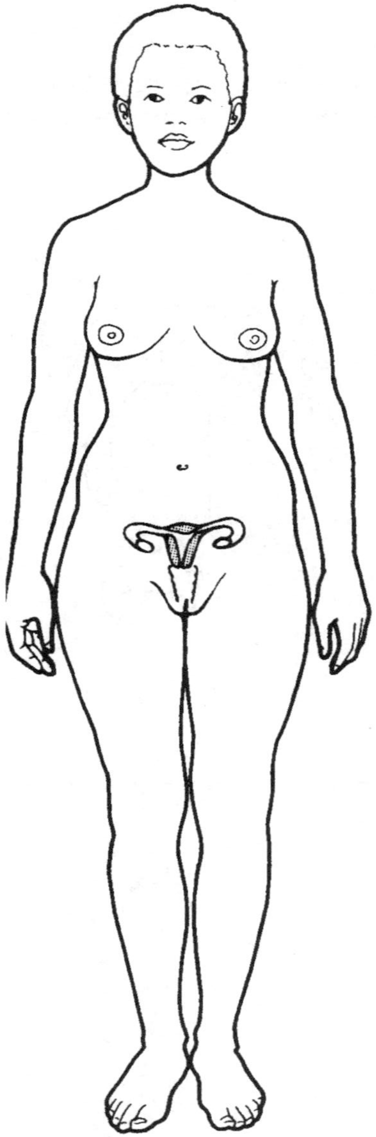

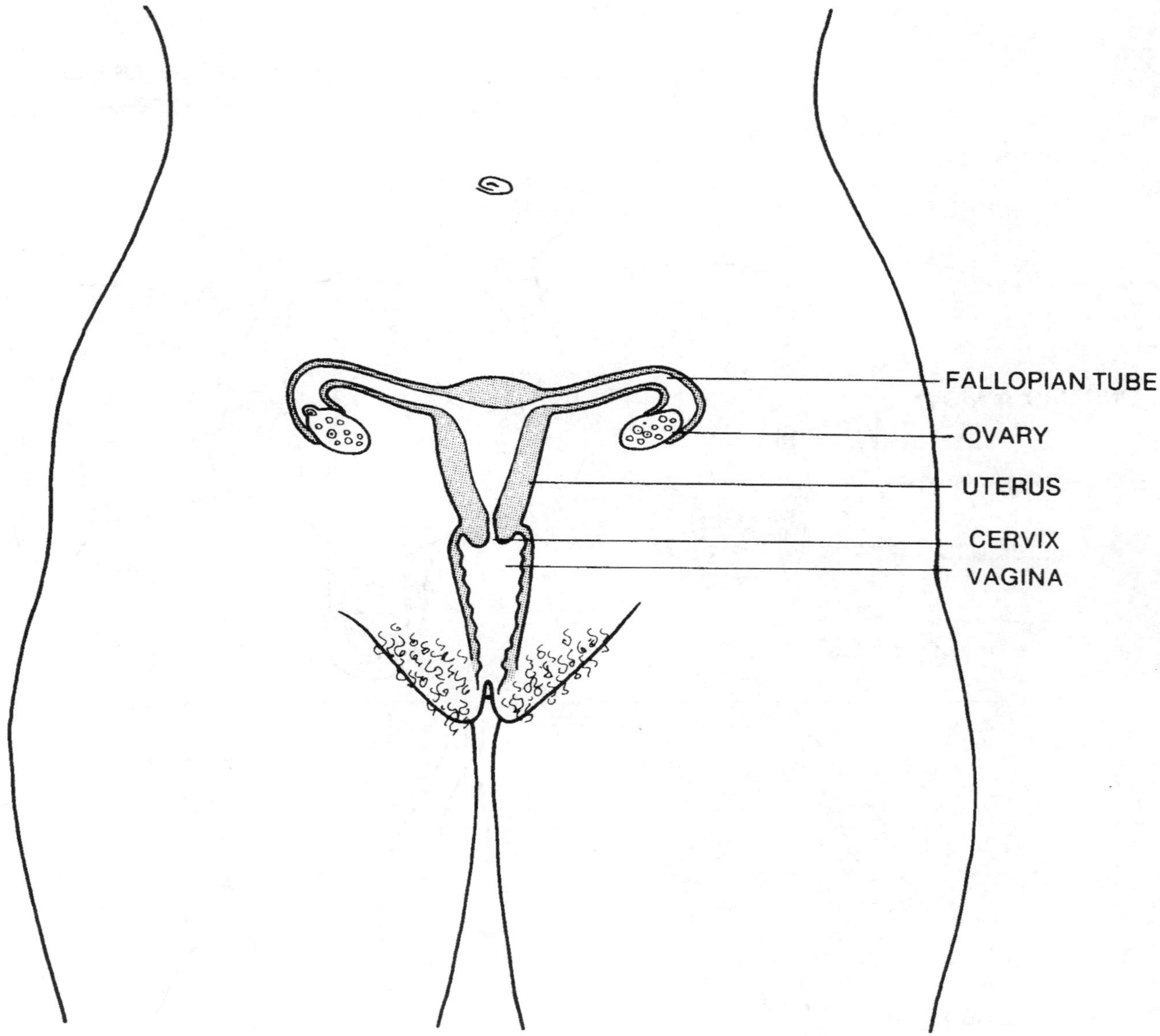

3. The internal (inner) reproductive organs (genital organs)

The internal, reproductive organs are the vagina, the uterus (womb), and the 2 ovaries (where egg cells are stored), which are connected by the 2 fallopian tubes.

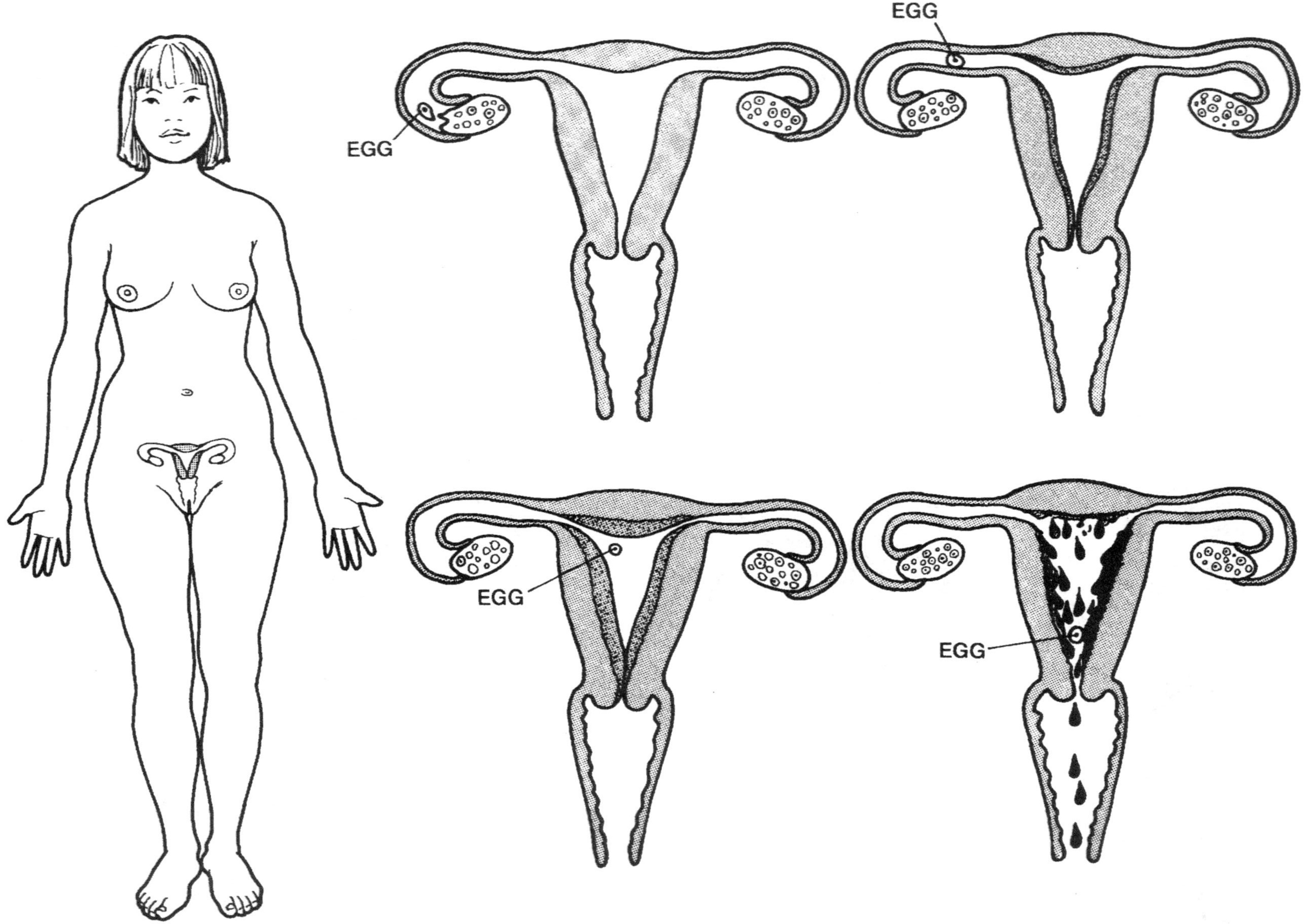

4. Menstruation

Menstruation is the monthly discharge of the blood-filled lining of the uterus (womb), and happens about every 4 weeks, if the female egg cell is not fertilized.

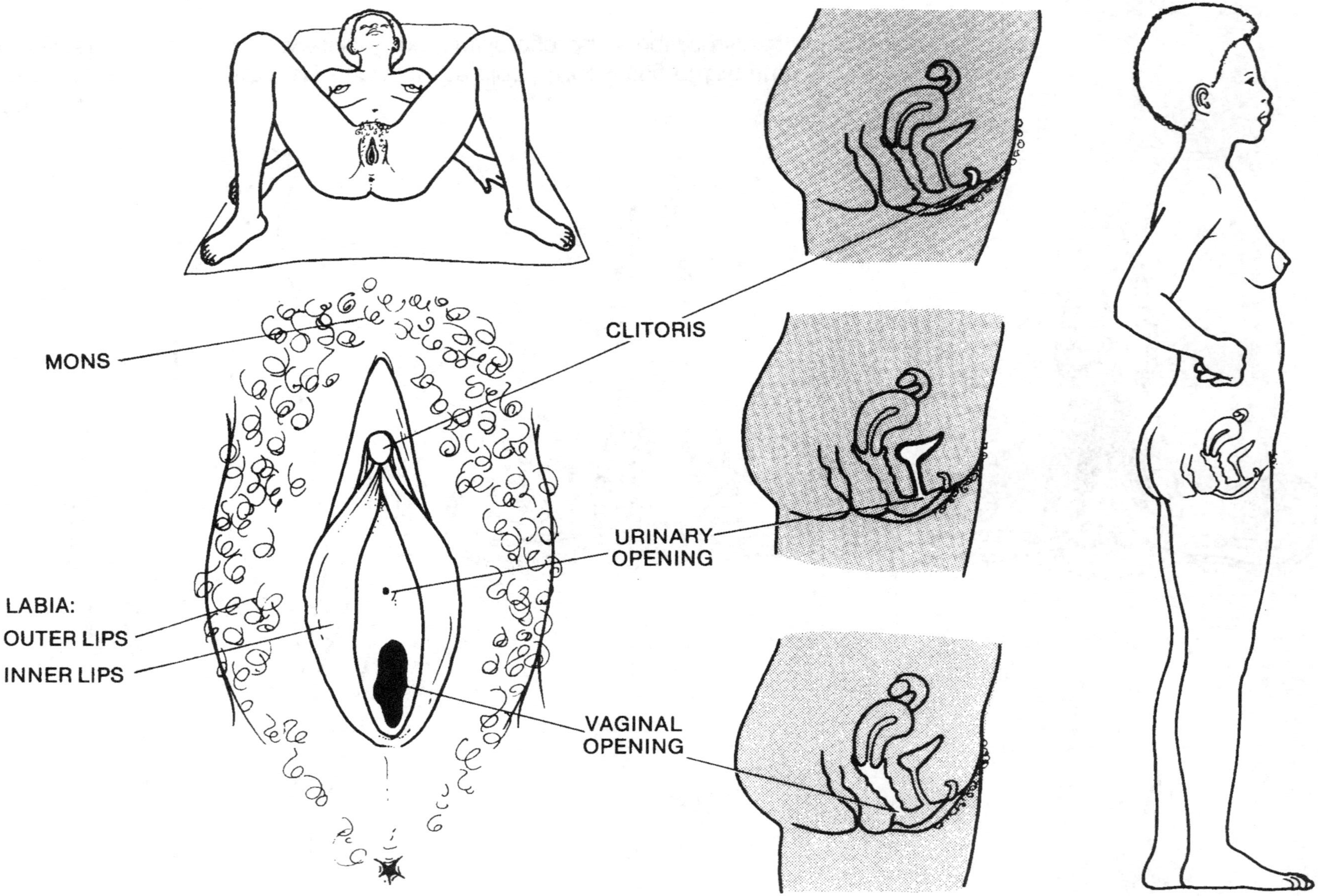

5. The external (outer) reproductive organs

All external reproductive or genital organs have important functions in a healthy woman's body. They are the outer lips (labia majora), the inner lips (labia minora), and the clitoris.

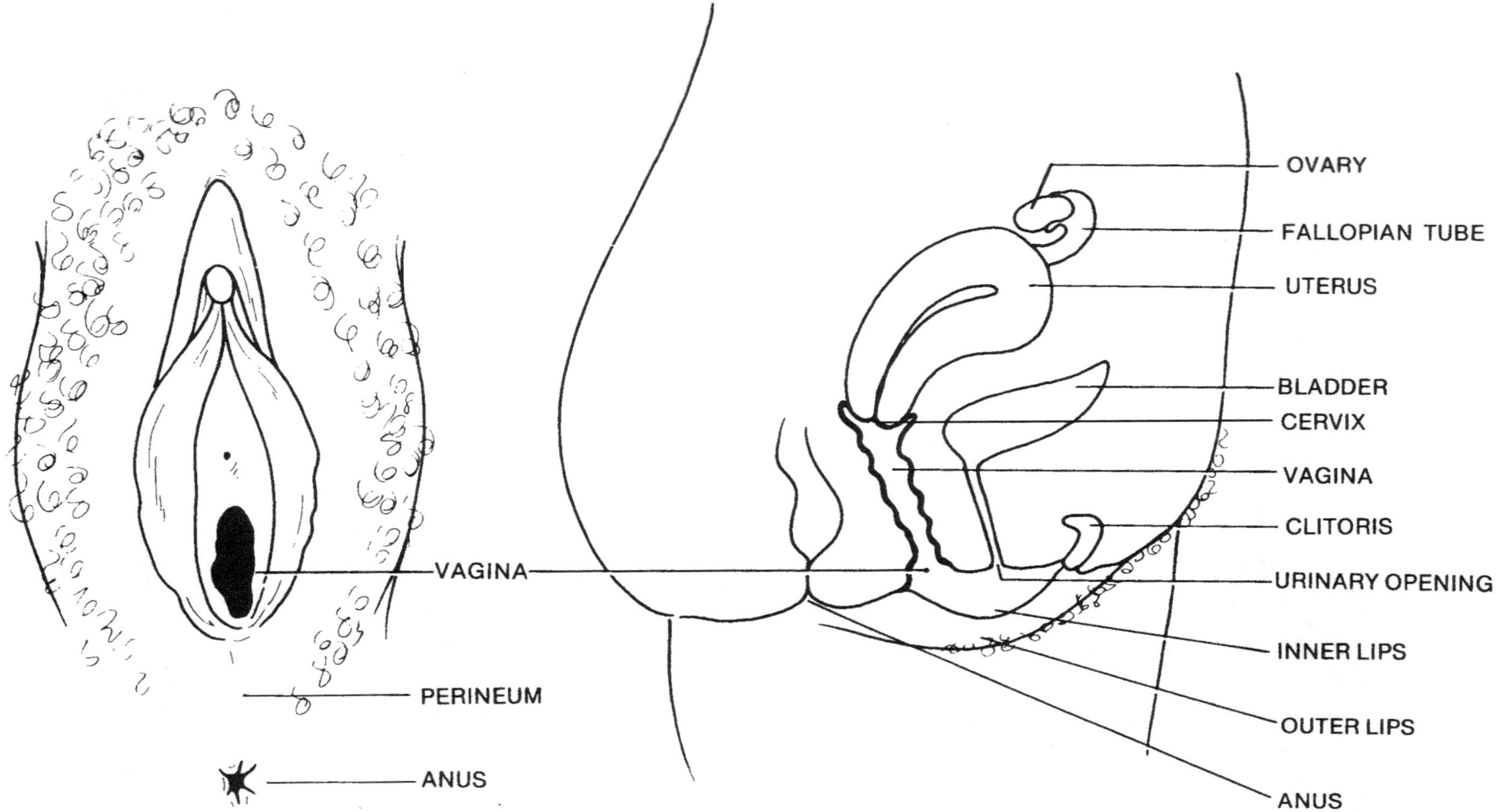

6. The external reproductive organs
The outer and inner lips protect the opening of the vagina and the clitoris.

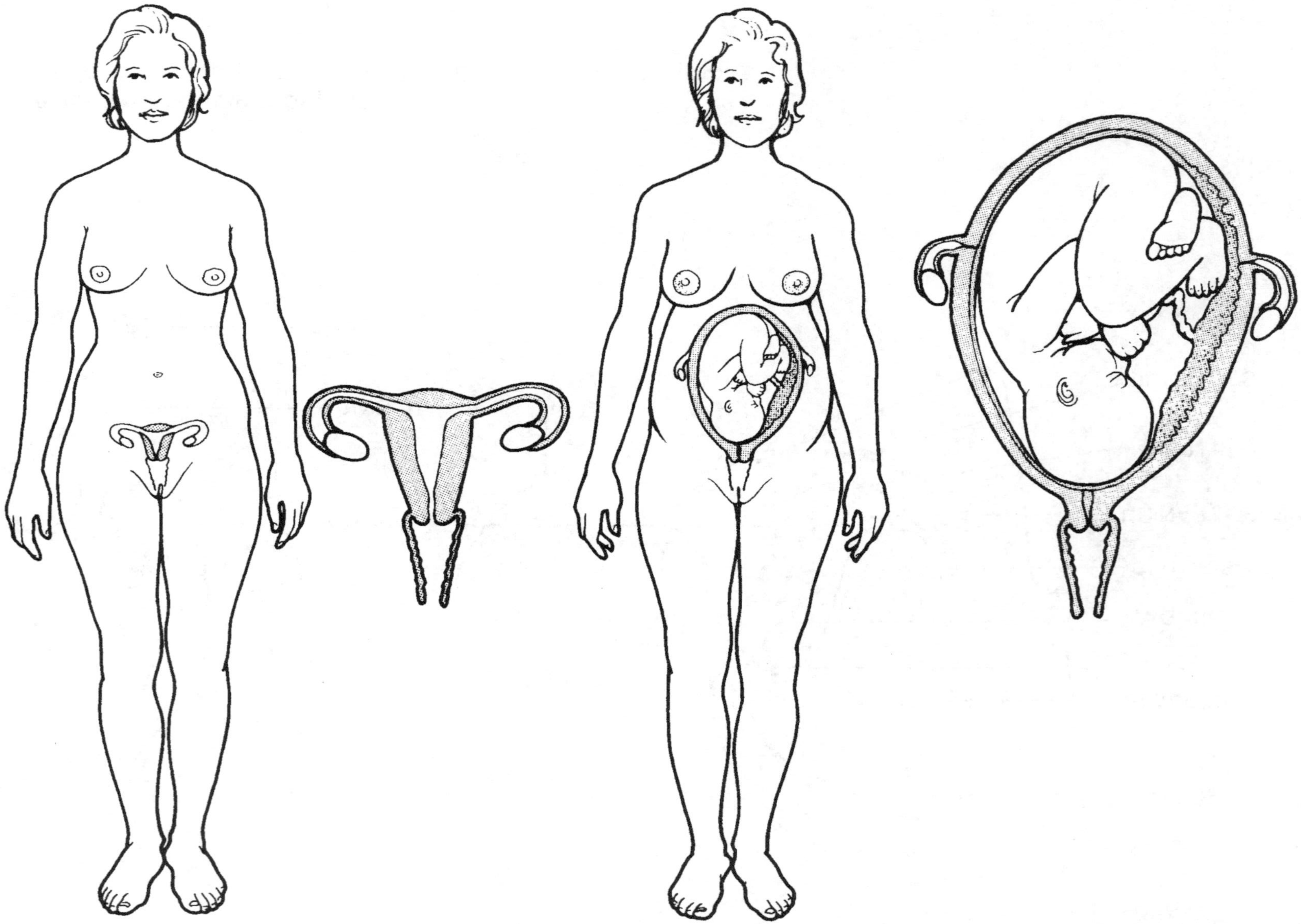

7. Body changes of pregnancy
We can see the changes of our bodies from pregnancy, inside and outside. The empty uterus is very different from the one with a baby inside.

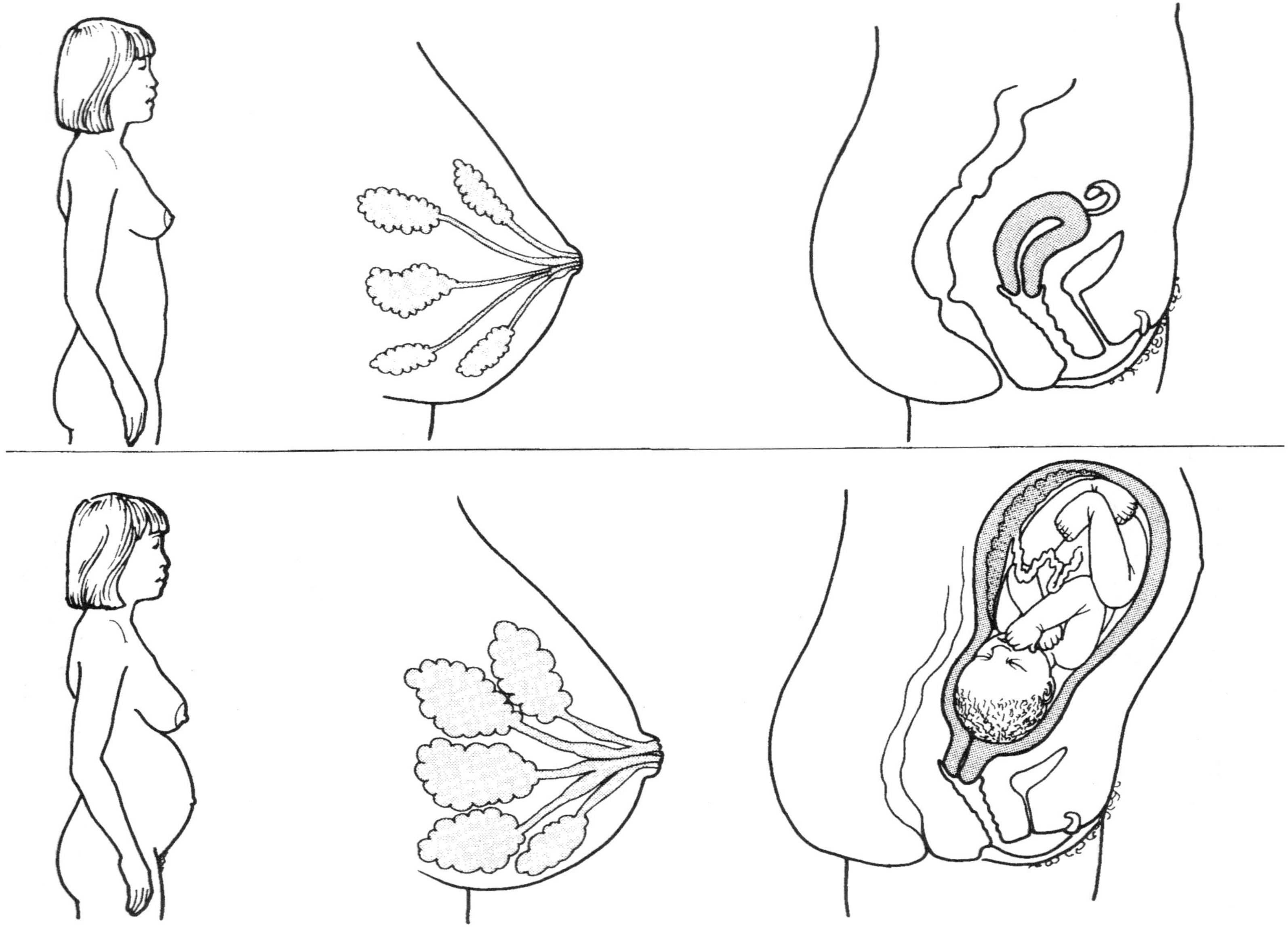

8. Body changes of pregnancy
Our bodies change on the outside as well as on the inside. We need special care during pregnancy.

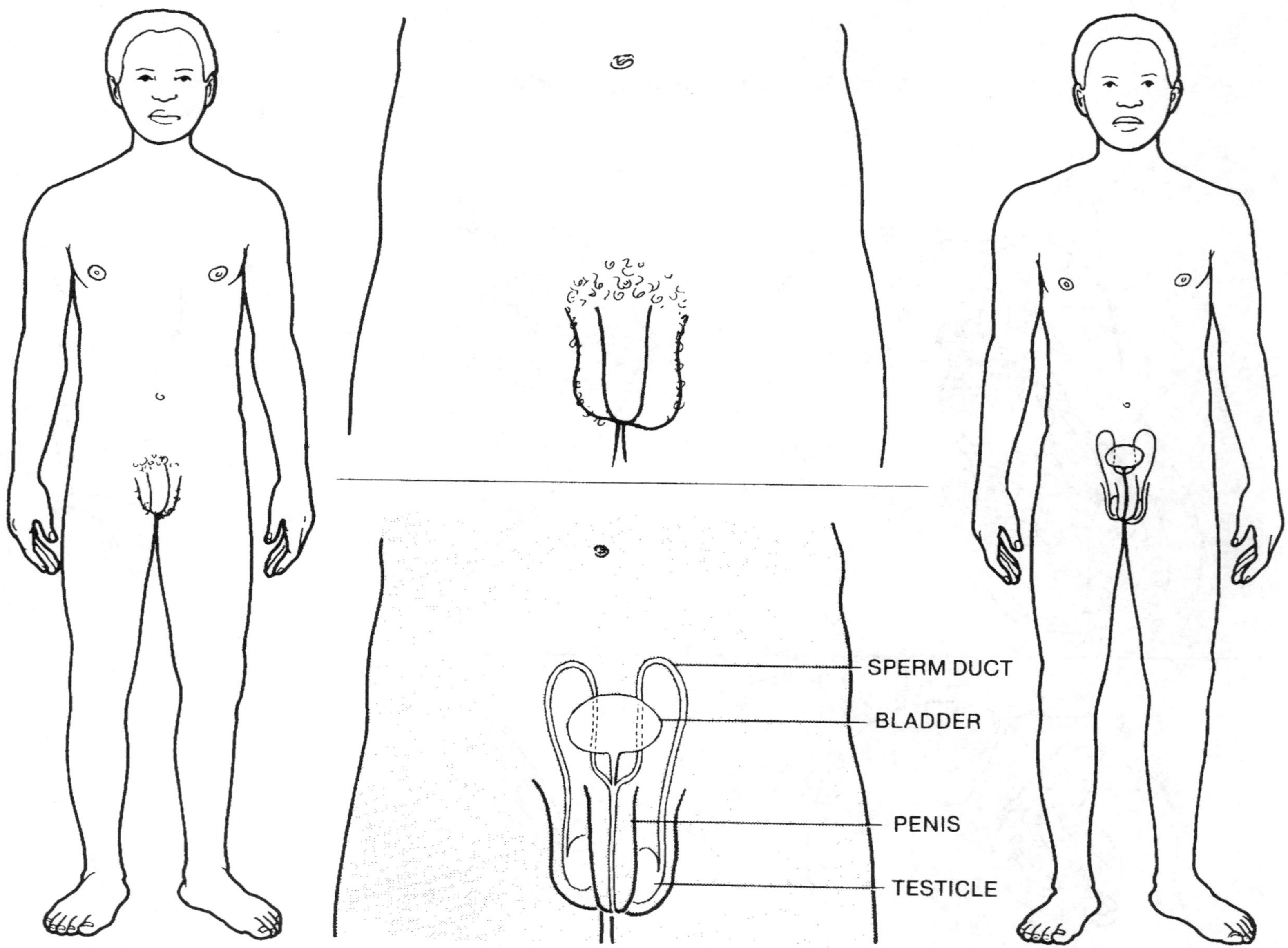

9. The male body and reproductive organs
The man's reproductive organs are mostly outside his body. They are the penis and the testicles. In the testicles, the sperm cells (male seeds) are made.

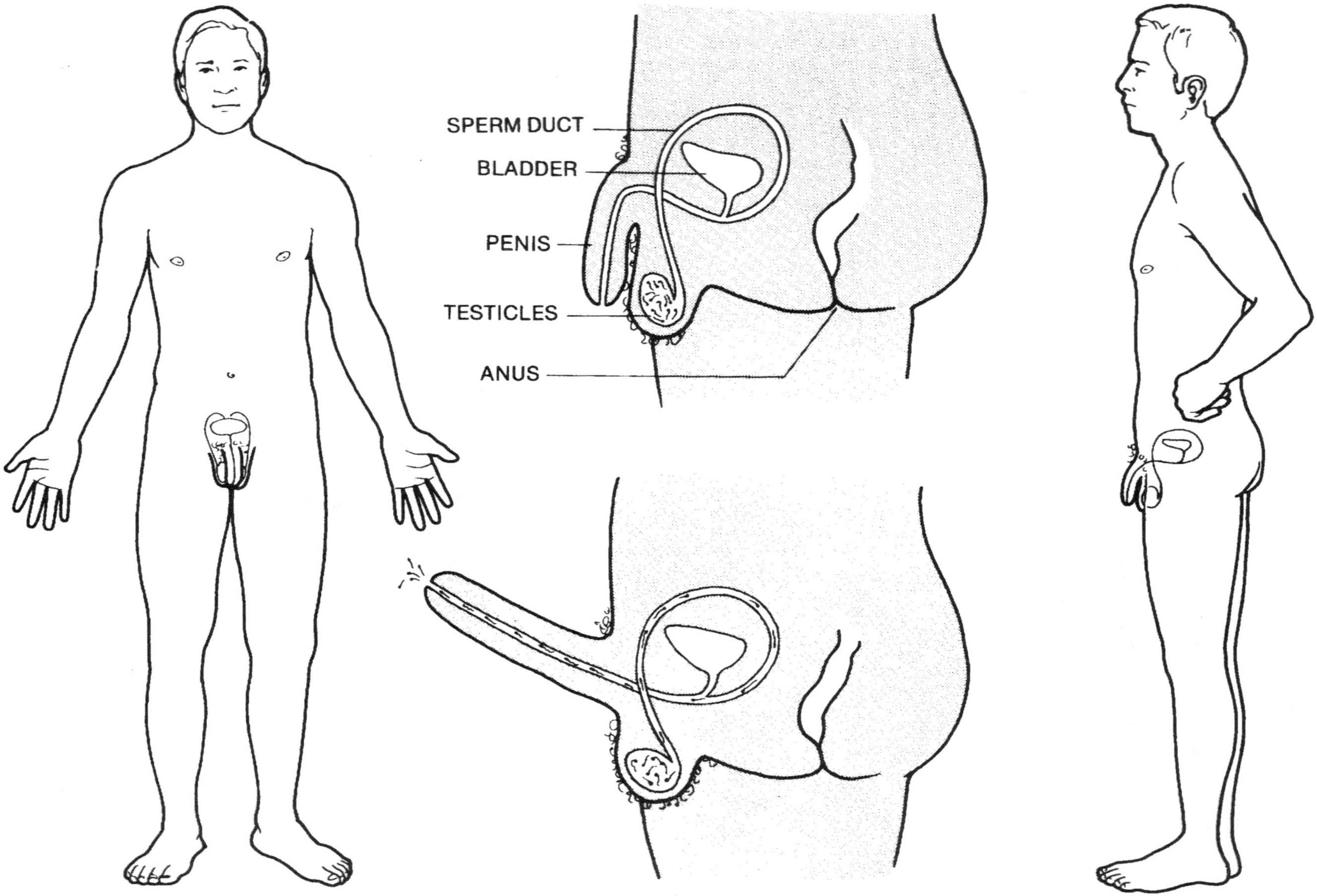

10. The male body and reproductive organs
The penis becomes hard and erect due to sexual excitement: then the sperm cells are squirted out in a liquid called semen.

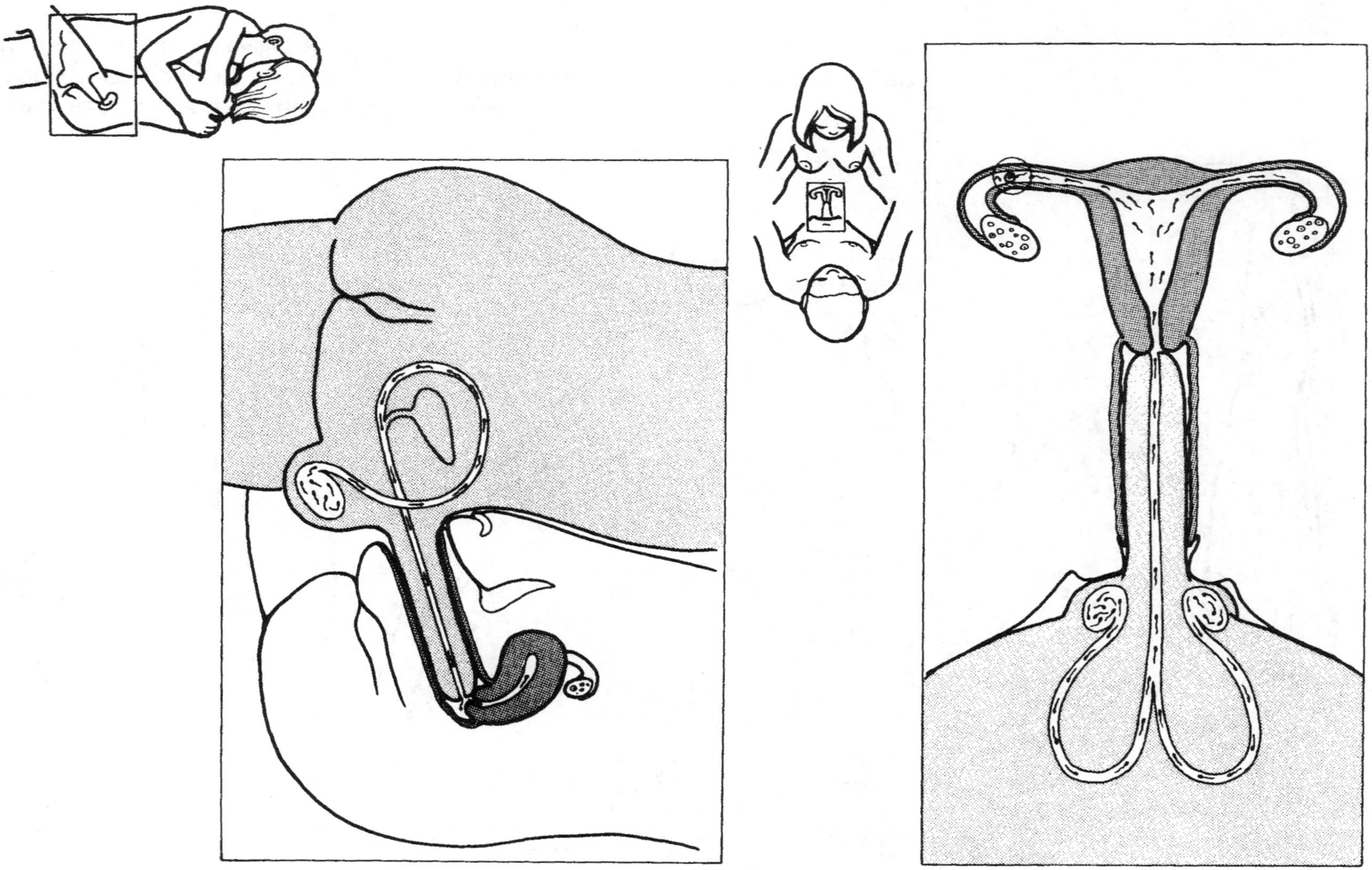

11. Fertilization

Millions of tiny sperm cells are put into the vagina by the penis during sexual intercourse. The sperm cells swim into the uterus and the Fallopian tubes. If they meet a ripe egg cell, it may be fertilized.

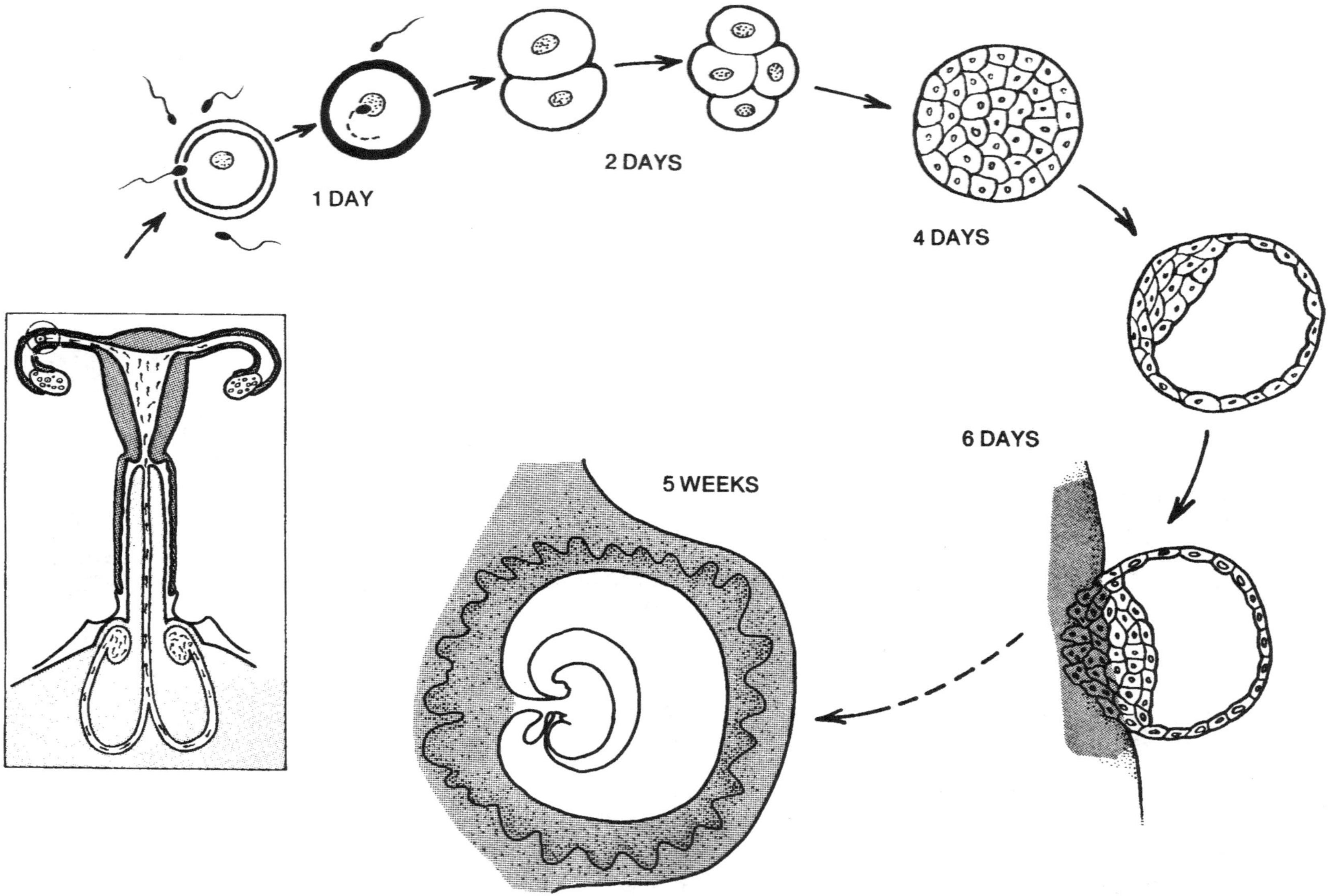

12. Fertilization

The ripe egg cell of a woman is fertilized when it is penetrated by a sperm cell of a man. Our most fertile time lasts several days, halfway between menstruations. The male sperm cell determines the sex of the future child at fertilization.

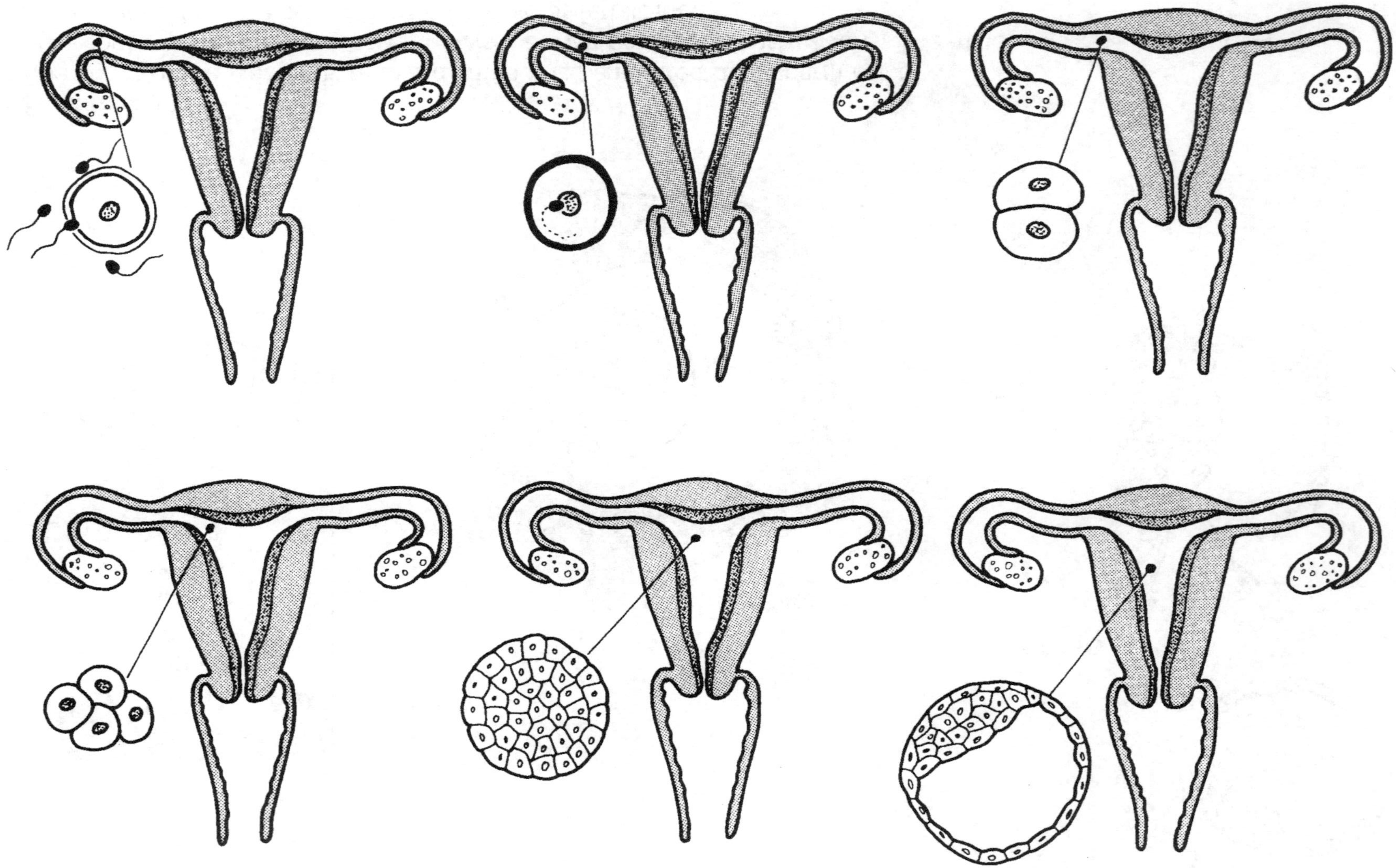

13. Fertilization and beginning of cell division
Only one sperm cell pushes through the outer wall of a ripe egg cell. The egg cell begins to divide and grow. The fertilized egg travels down the Fallopian tube to the uterus.

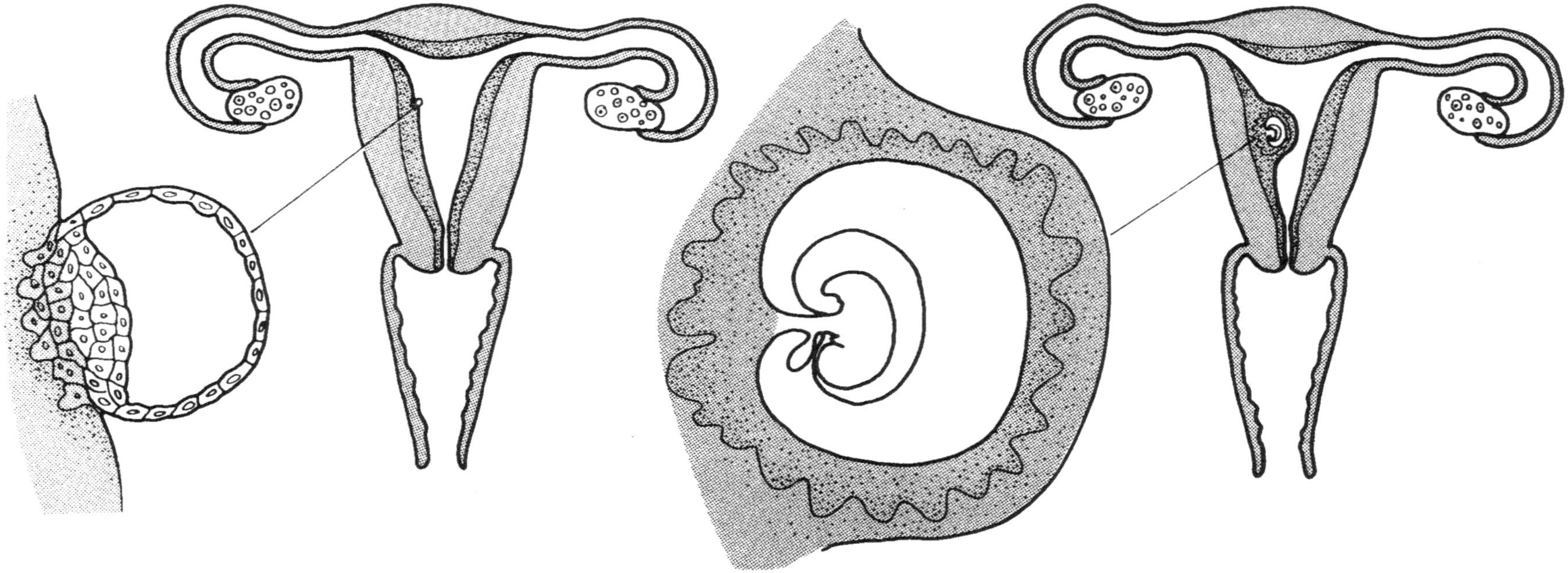

14. Implantation and beginning of growth

The fertilized egg cell moves from the Fallopian tube into the uterus. There, attached to the soft lining, it grows quickly. It is much too small to see.

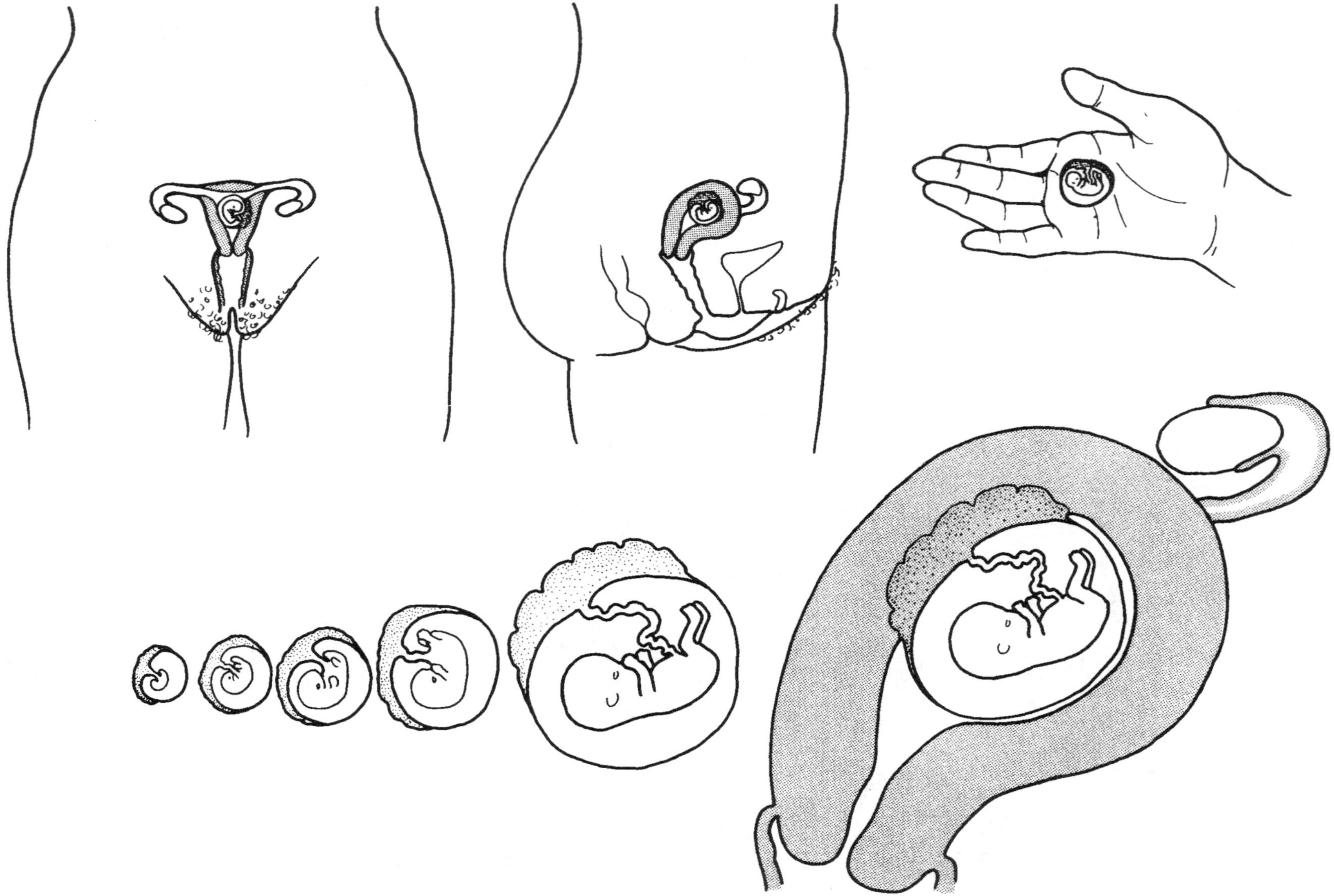

15. Development of the embryo: The first 3 months
It takes 3 months for the fertilized egg cell to form an embryo inside a sac filled with fluid. This sac is inside the uterus.

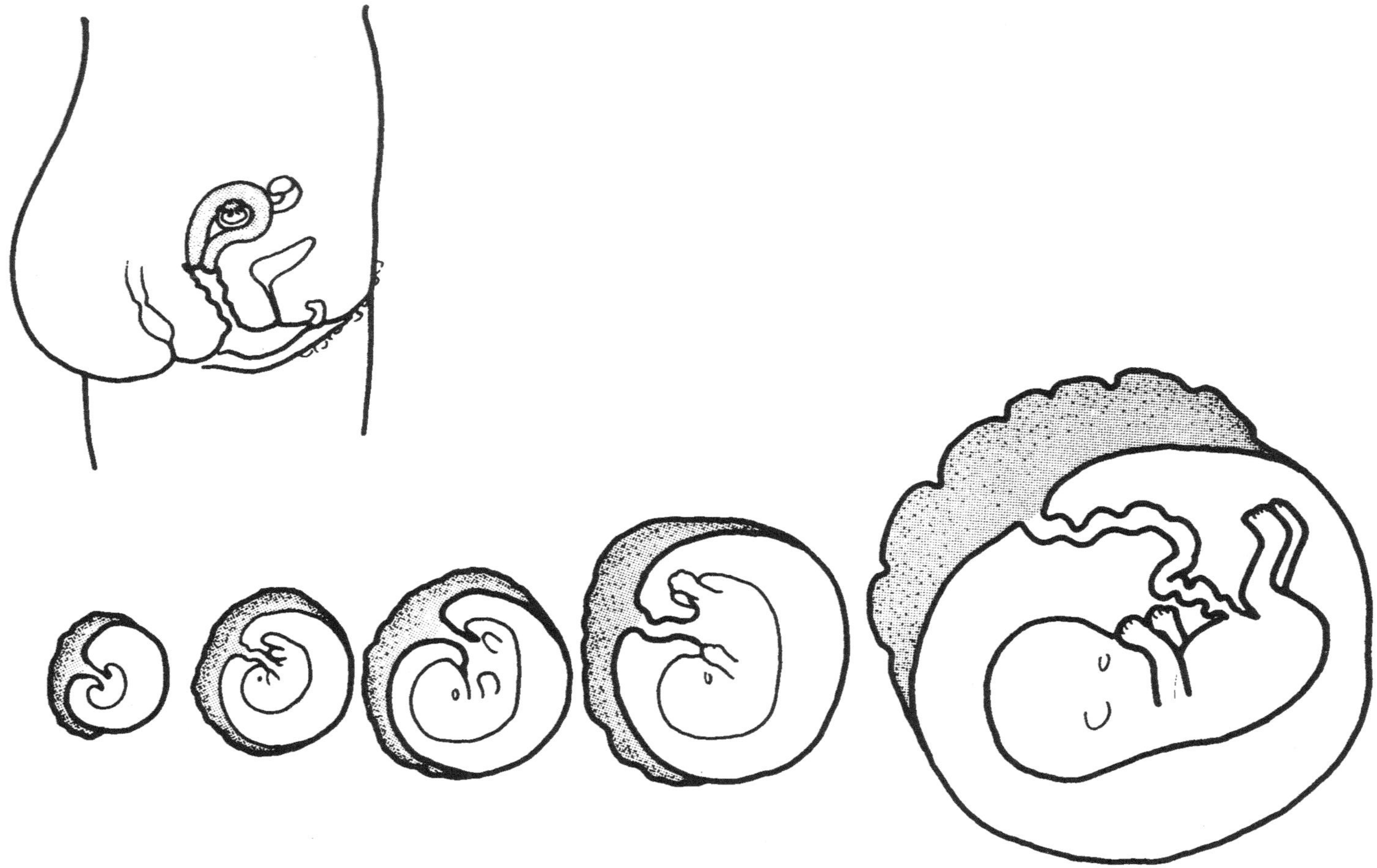

16. Development of the embryo: The first 3 months

The embryo first develops the head and spine. It is connected by the umbilical cord to the placenta for food, oxygen, and removal of waste. Our body makes the placenta.

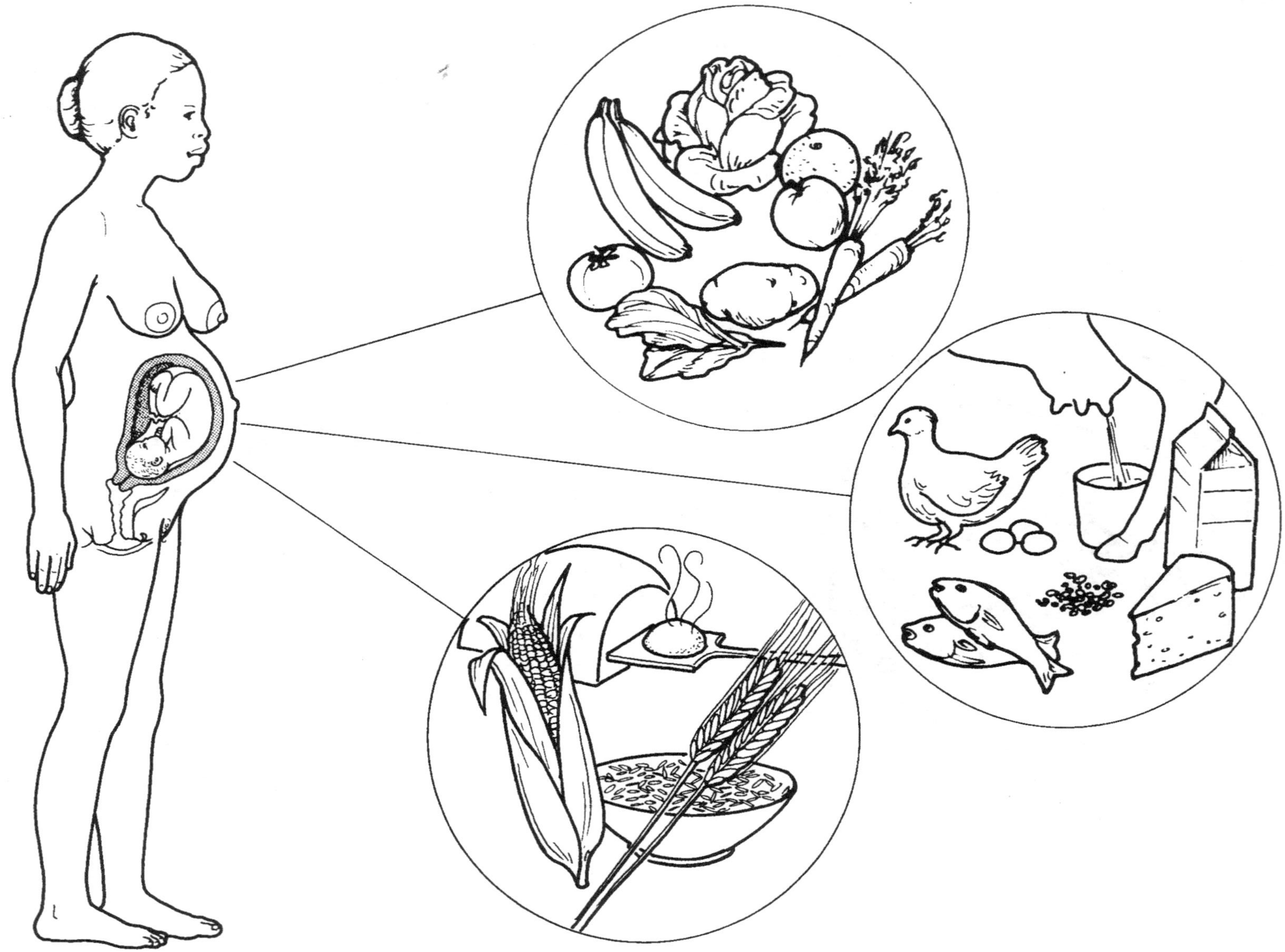

17. The food we need

To grow a healthy baby, we must eat enough and also all kinds of different foods, including meat, fish, eggs, all kinds of vegetables, fruits, bread and cereals, and drink lots of fluids.

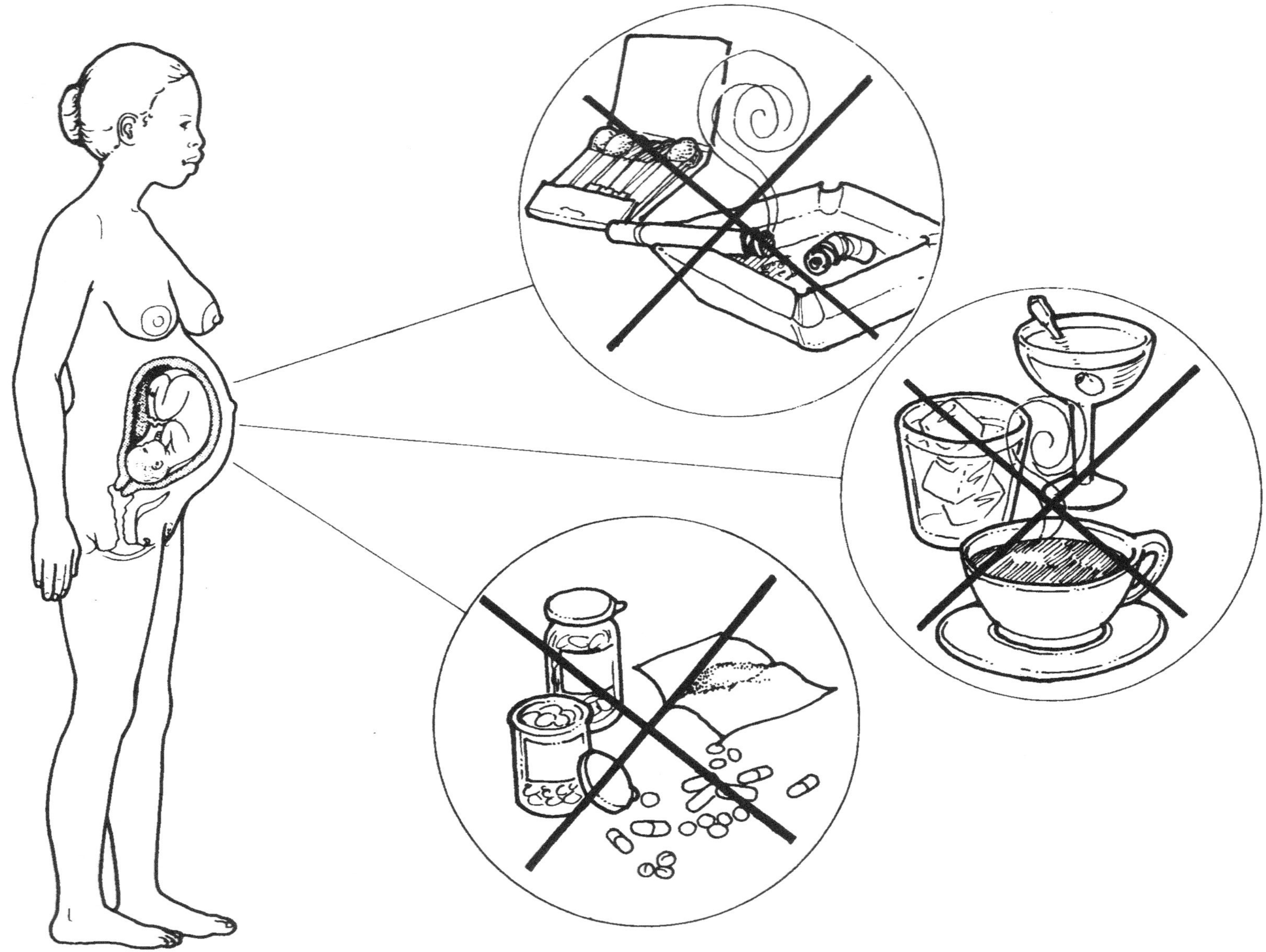

18. What to avoid

The growth and health of the baby depends on what we eat and drink during pregnancy. Alcohol, cigarettes, and drugs are bad for the mother's health, and dangerous for the baby during pregnancy.

TO THE TEACHER / GROUP LEADER:

PLEASE PREPARE SOME DRAWINGS AND PICTURES (CLIPPINGS FROM MAGAZINES) OF THE MOST COMMON LOCAL FOODS AND DISHES, AND PASTE THEM ON THIS PAGE (COVERING UP THIS MESSAGE). THE PICTURES SHOULD SHOW A COMBINATION OF FOODS THAT MAKE A BALANCED MEAL WHERE YOU TEACH/LIVE. PLEASE CONSIDER COSTS AND AVAILABILITY IN THE MAKE-UP OF THE DISHES/MEALS AND OUTLINE THE BASIC COSTS OF BALANCED MEALS.

THE AIM IS TO SHOW ON THIS PAGE THOSE LOCALLY AVAILABLE, INEXPENSIVE FOODS THAT MAKE A BALANCED DIET: SUCH A BALANCED MEAL SHOULD INCLUDE ALL THE IMPORTANT FOOD VALUES DISCUSSED IN PICTURE 17.

19. Familiar foods we know and eat
These familiar foods, eaten regularly — every week — make a balanced diet.

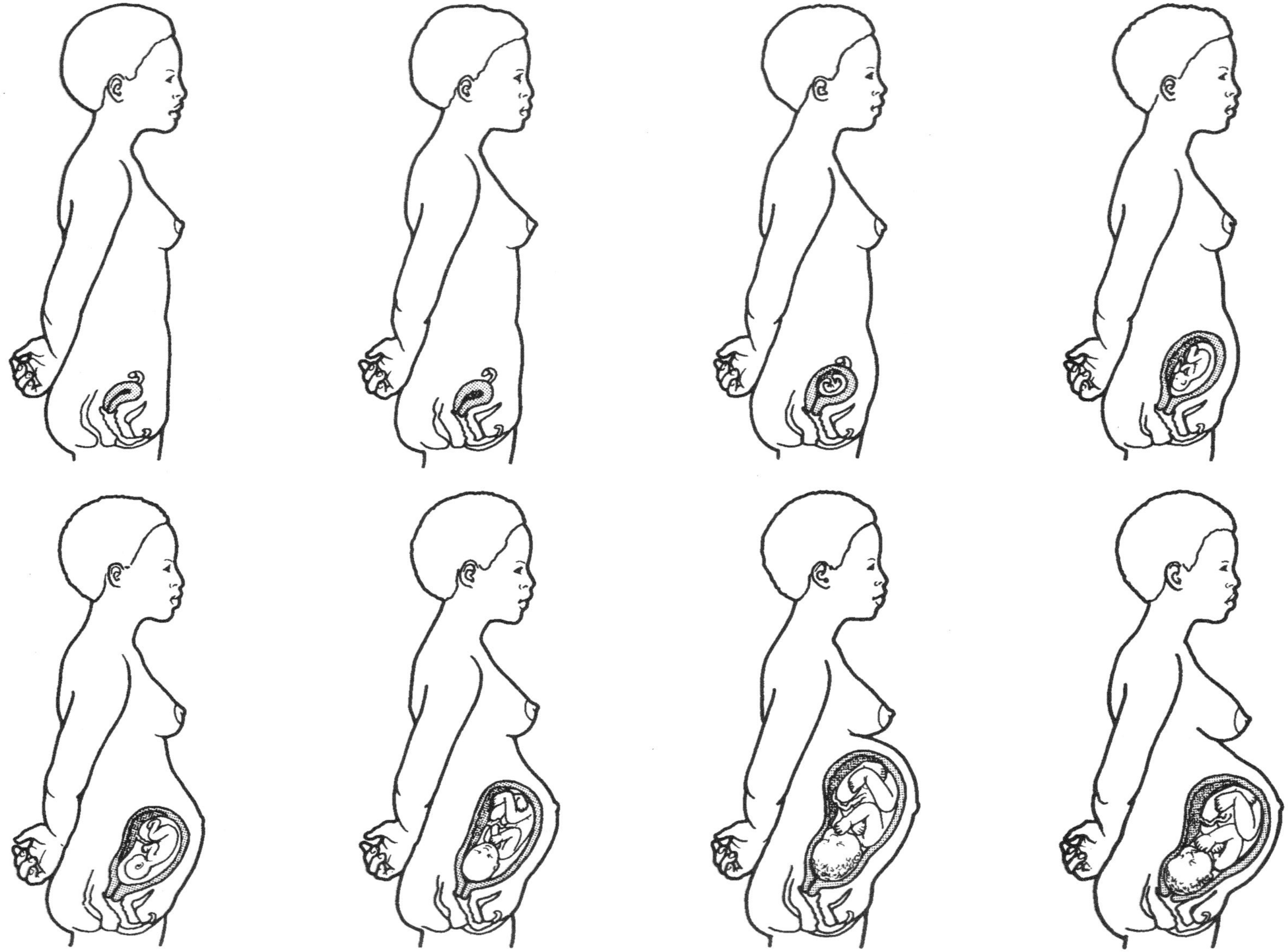

20. The development of the pregnancy
Inside the uterus, the tiny fertilized egg cell grows. During the first 6 months of pregnancy (see top row) our appearance changes very little. During the last 3 months (bottom row) many changes happen that we can see.

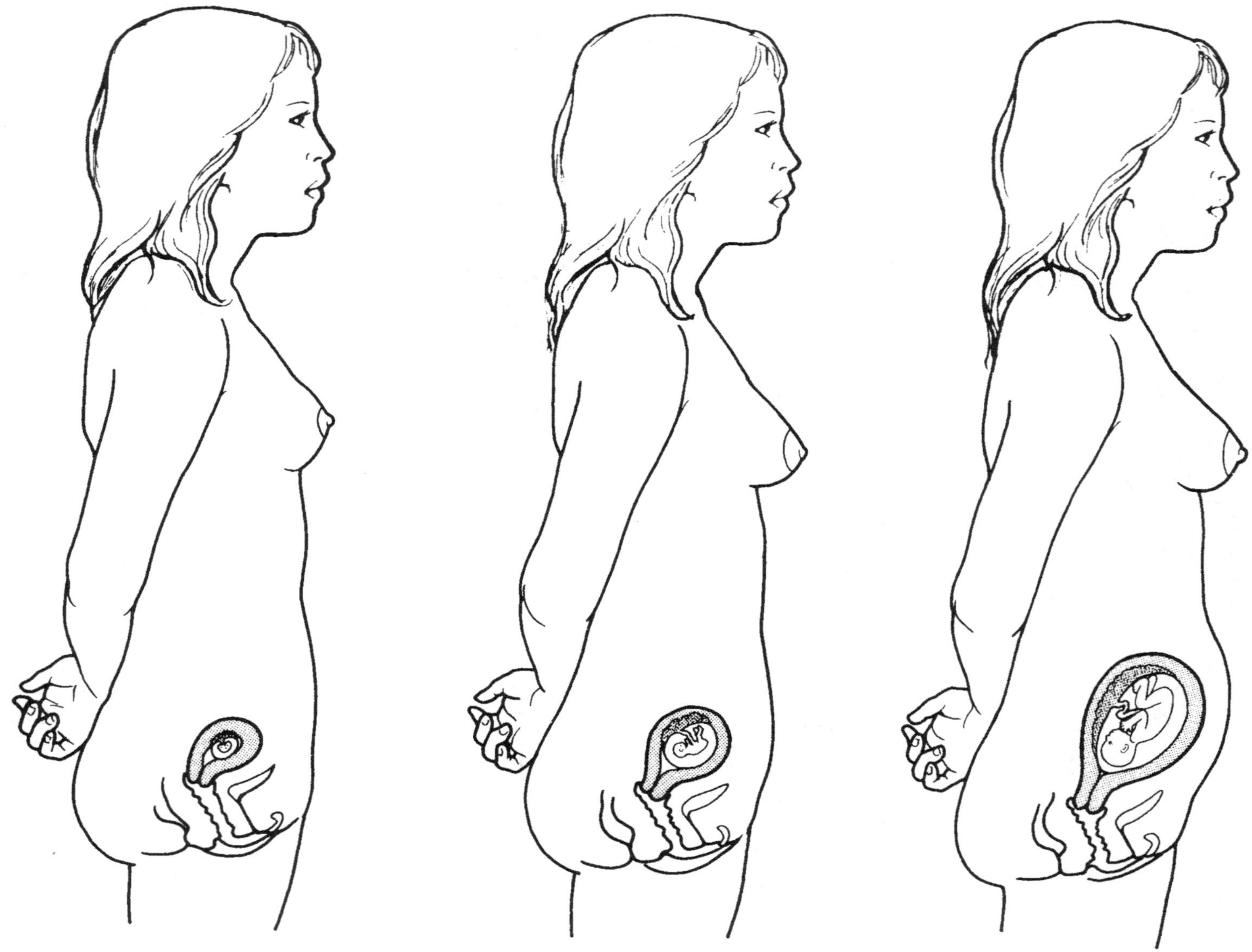

21. The development of the pregnancy
After 3 months the embryo is called a "fetus". At mid-pregnancy we begin to feel the fetus move. Our breasts also get bigger in preparation for making milk. No special care is needed for the breasts.

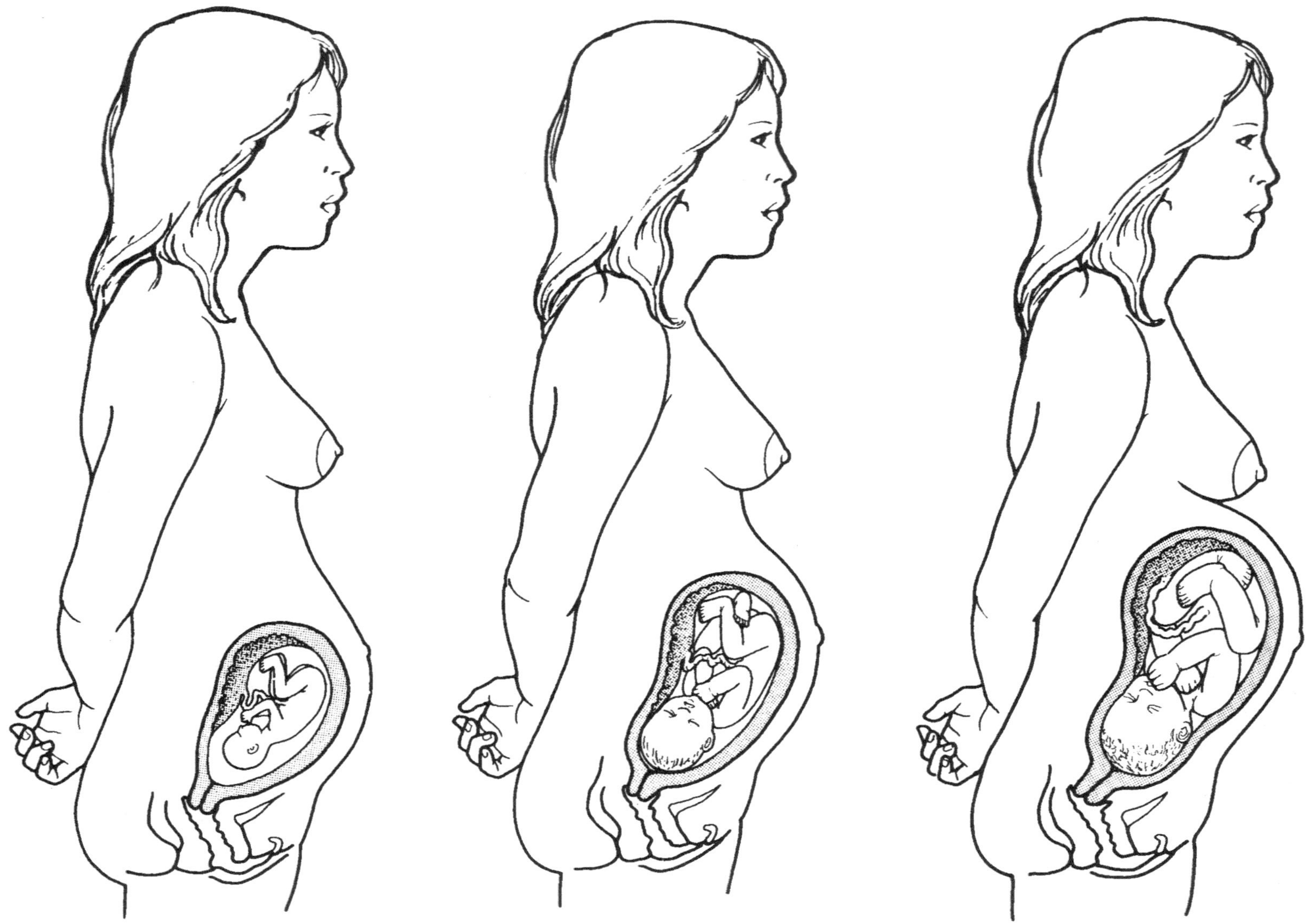

22. The development of the pregnancy
During the last 3 months, the fetus gets bigger very quickly and so does our body.

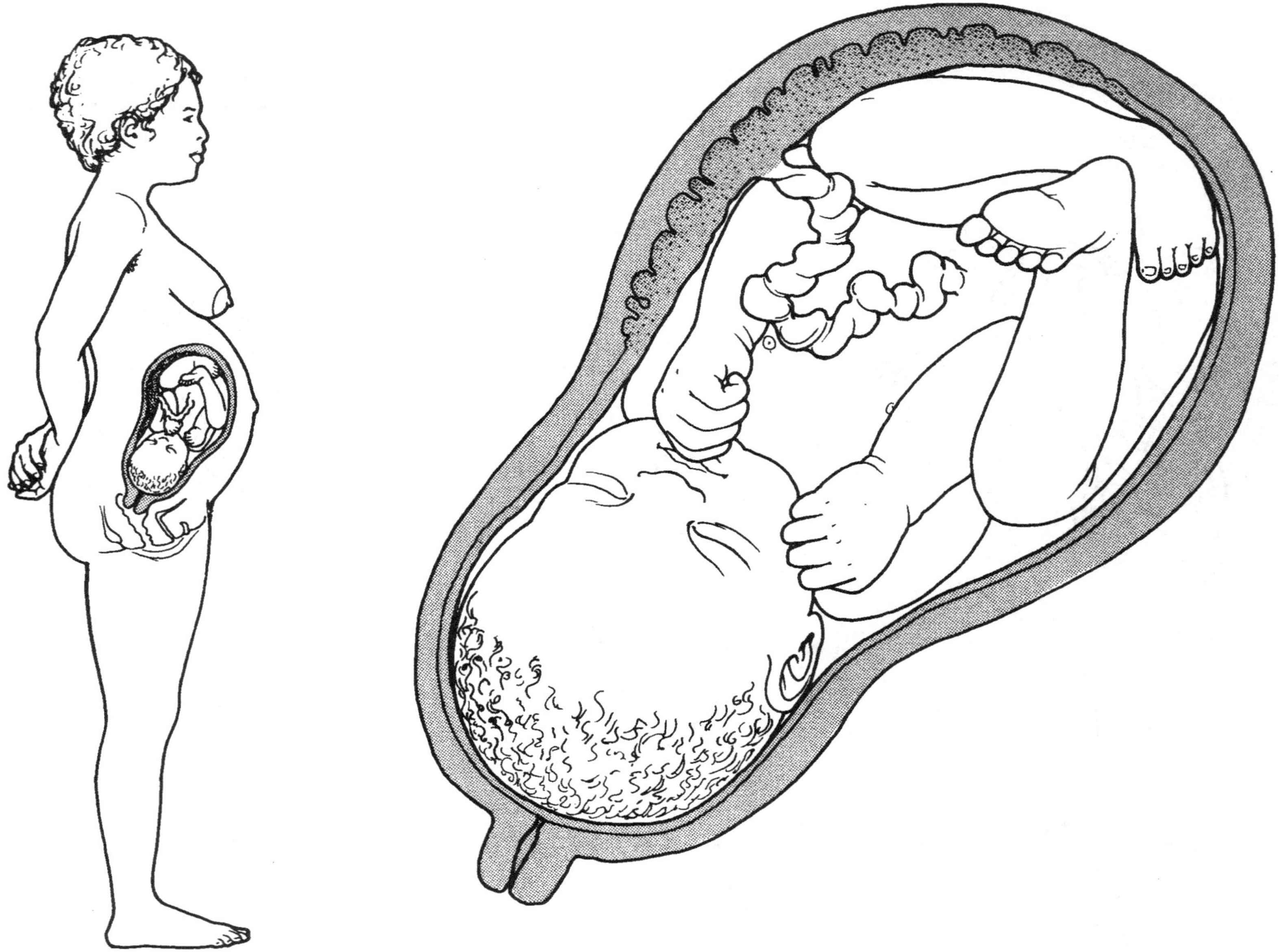

23. Just before birth

At 9 months the fetus has become a fully- developed baby. It is now ready to live outside our body.

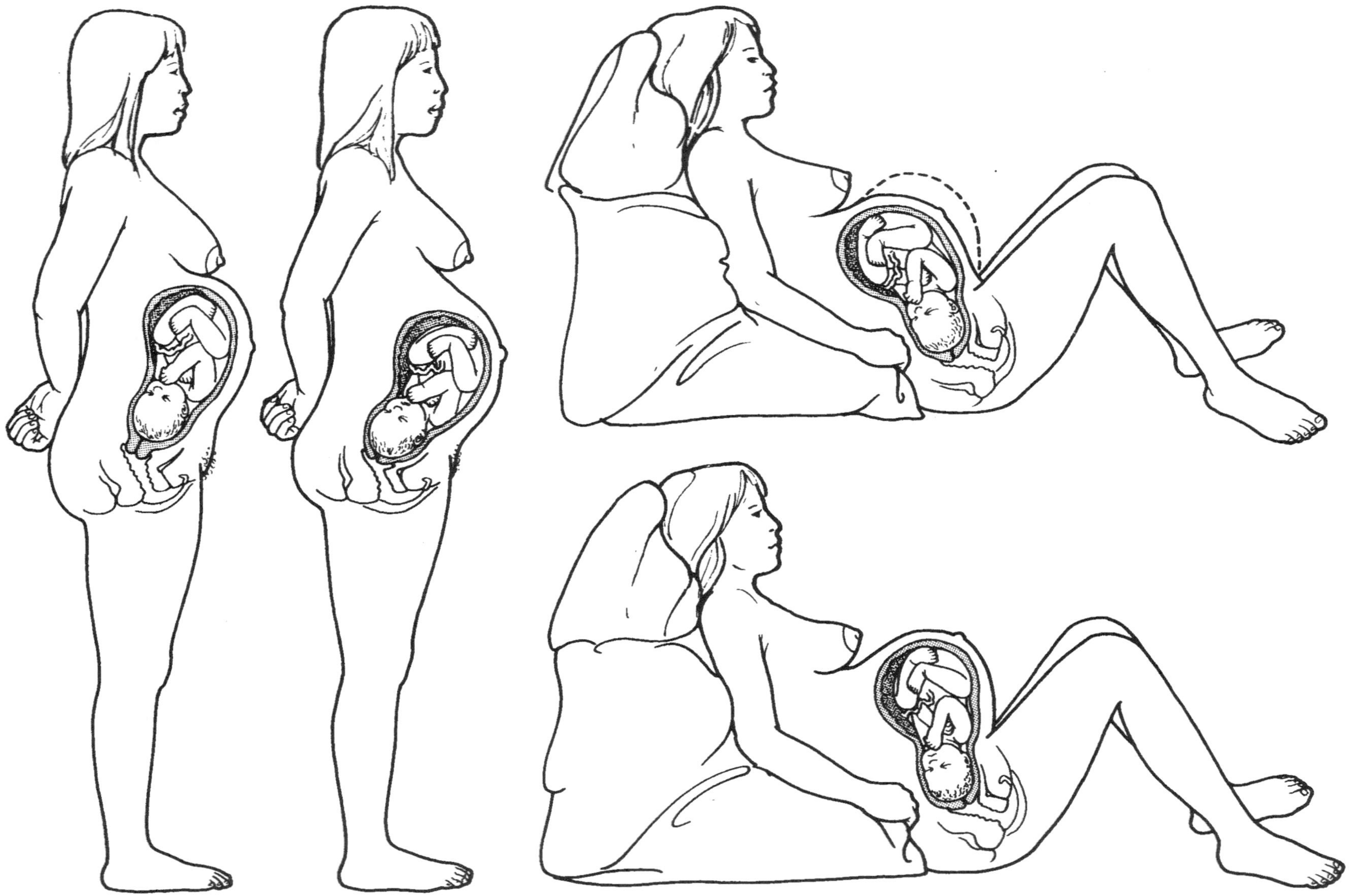

24. The beginning of labor
The fetus moves into position just before labor begins. The labor pains or contractions open the uterus and push the baby out through the vagina. The sac in which the fetus has developed breaks, and the fluid comes out.

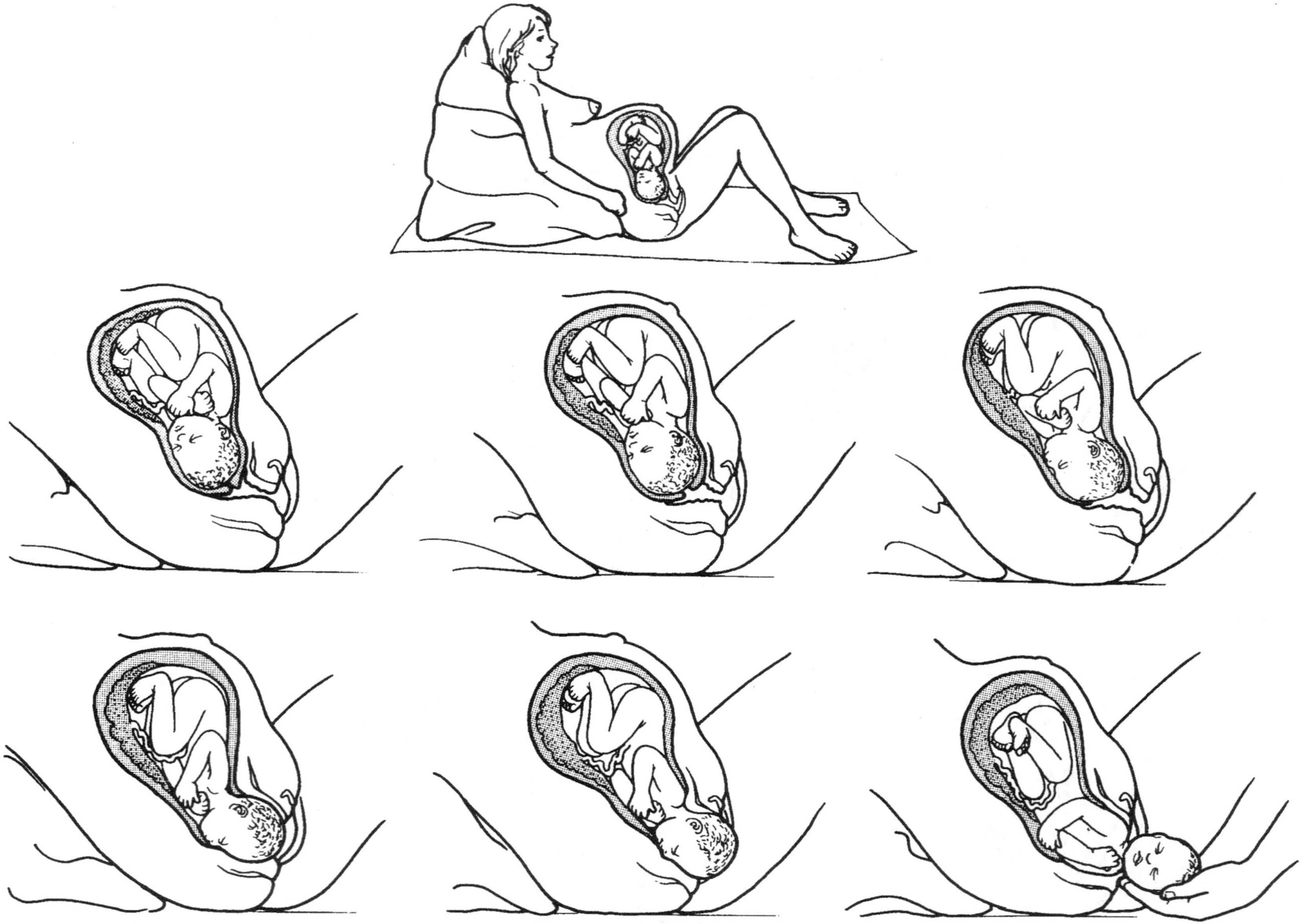

25. The birth process

Birth starts with the opening (dilation) of the cervix — the door to the uterus. Then the baby is pushed into the birth canal and out through the stretching skinfolds of the vagina.

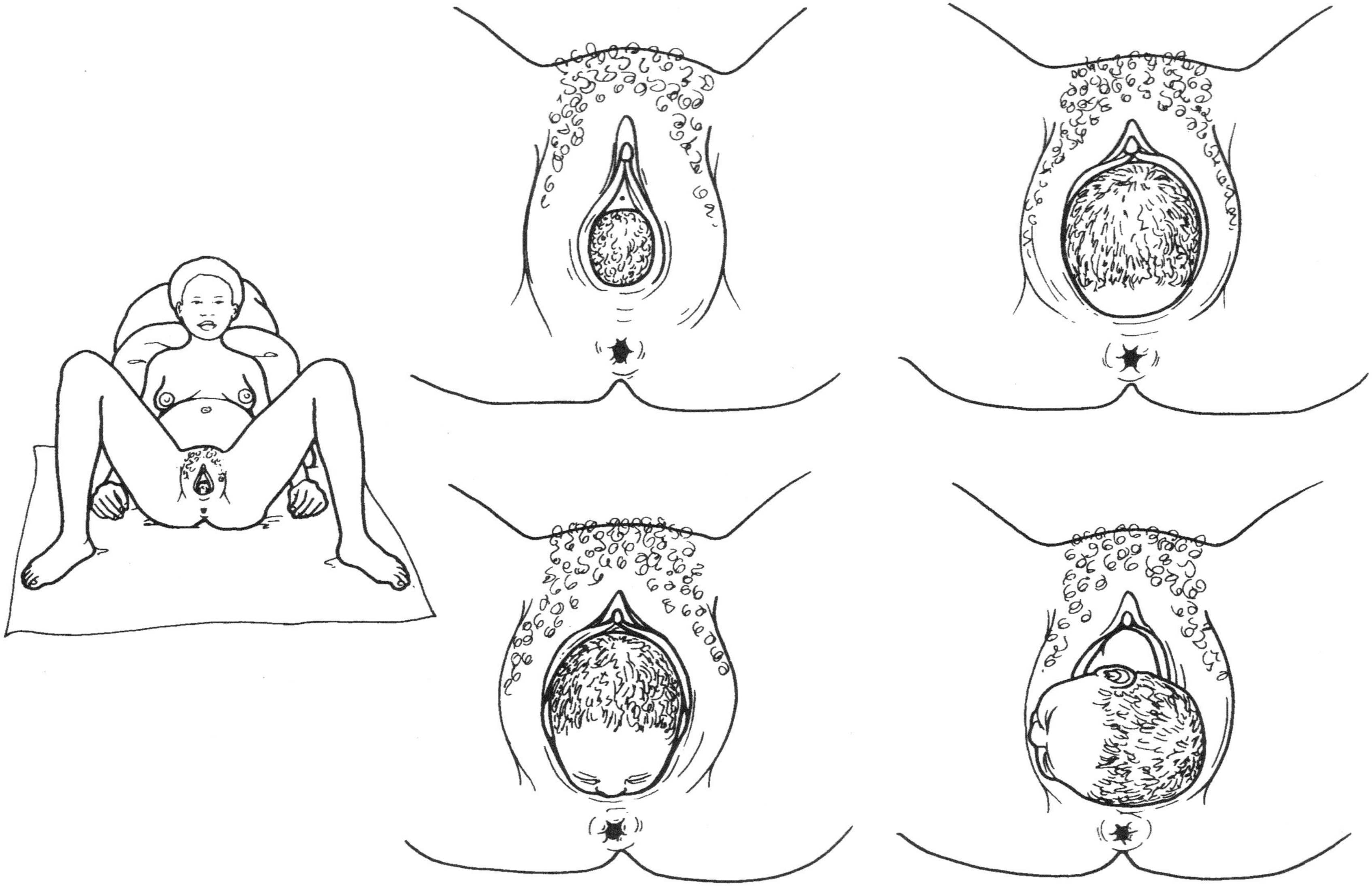

26. The birth process
Seen from the outside, the baby's head comes out by turning through the elastic opening of the vagina. The skinfolds are soft and stretch without harming the baby's head.

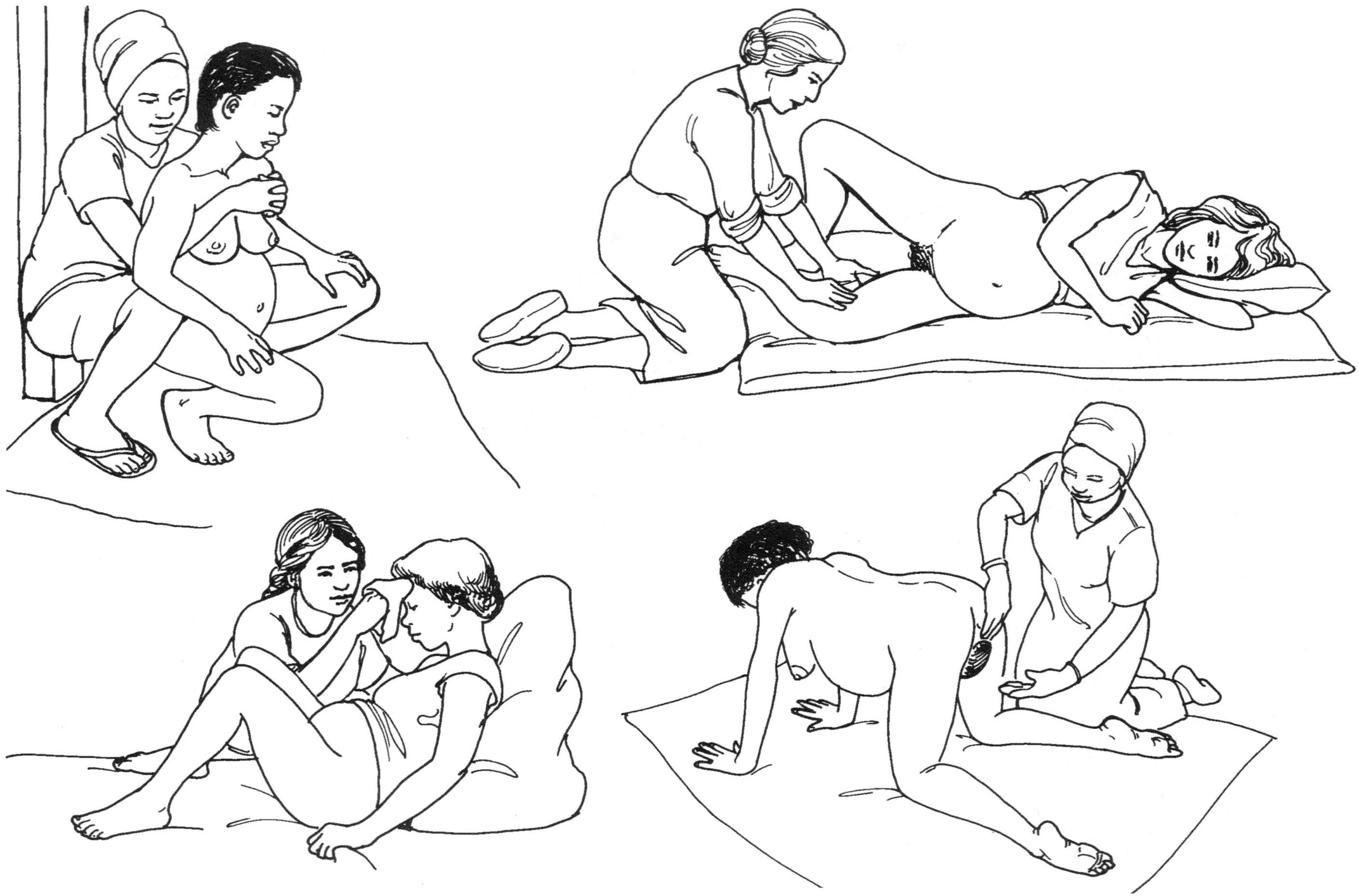

27. Birth positions of mothers

Women around the world give birth in many different positions. It is easier to push the baby down than up. Use the position that is most comfortable for you. Giving birth is hard work: we need extra support and encouragement at this time.

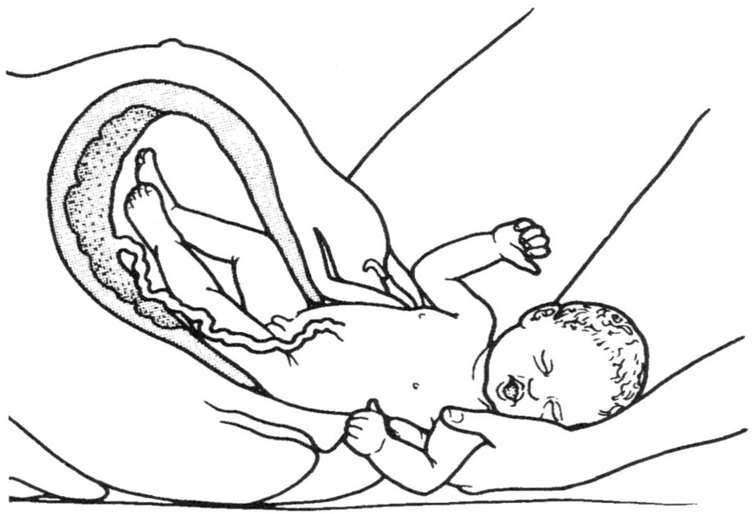

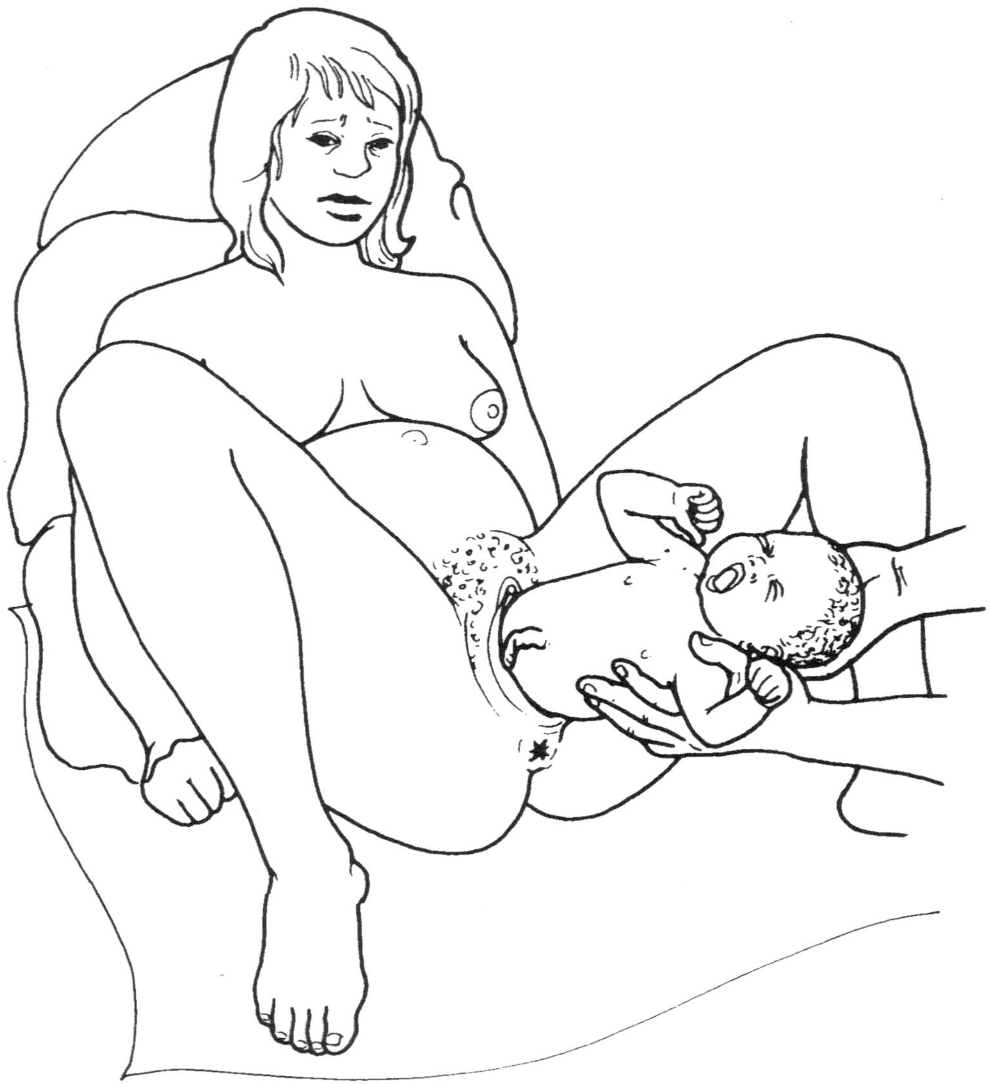

28. Birth

Birth takes hard work, patience and time. A newborn baby usually starts breathing and crying right away. The mucus should be cleared from its nose and throat. If the baby does not breathe, mouth-to-mouth resuscitation must be given at once.

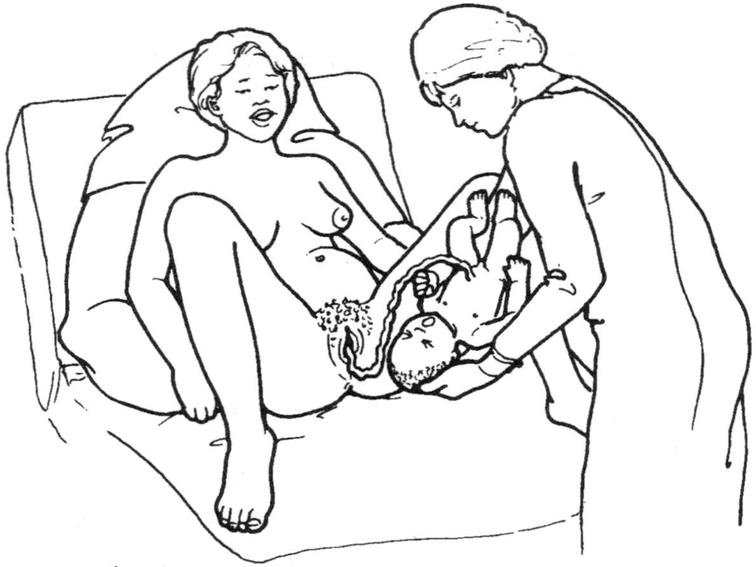

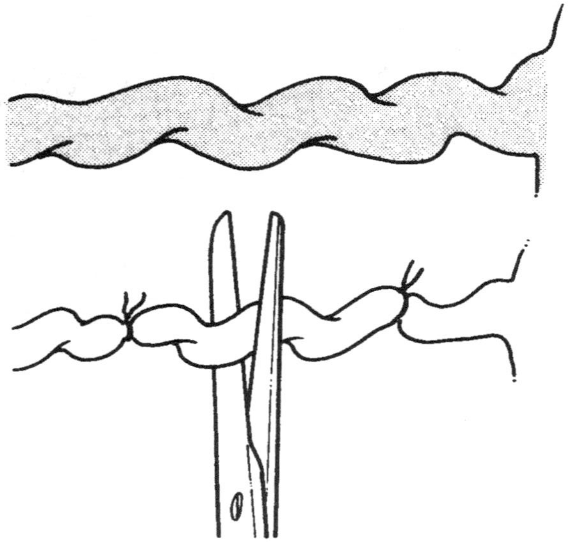

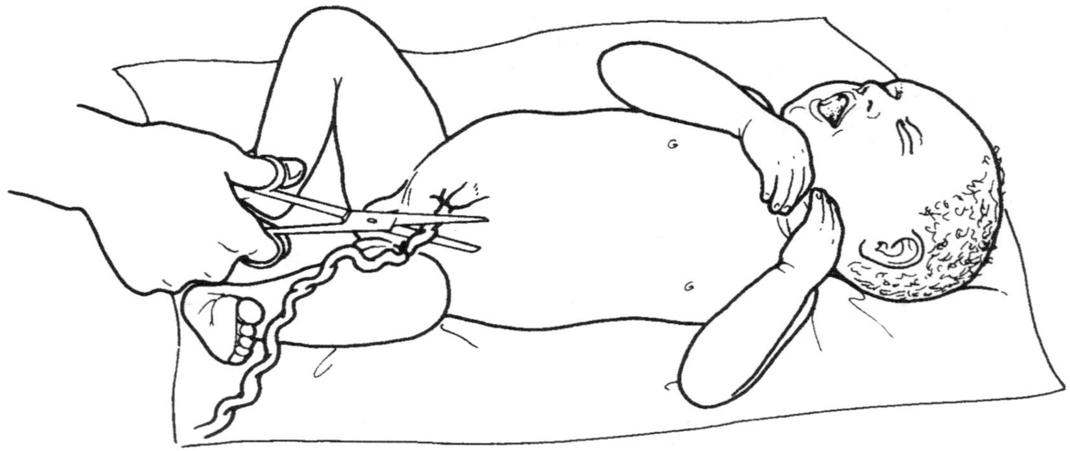

29. Immediate newborn care

After the baby is born, and the cord has stopped pulsating, the cord is tied in 2 places. Then the cord is cut with a sterile instrument between the 2 ties. The stump should be left alone to dry. The newborn should be given to the mother or placed on her abdomen at birth. This is the warmest and safest place for the baby to be.

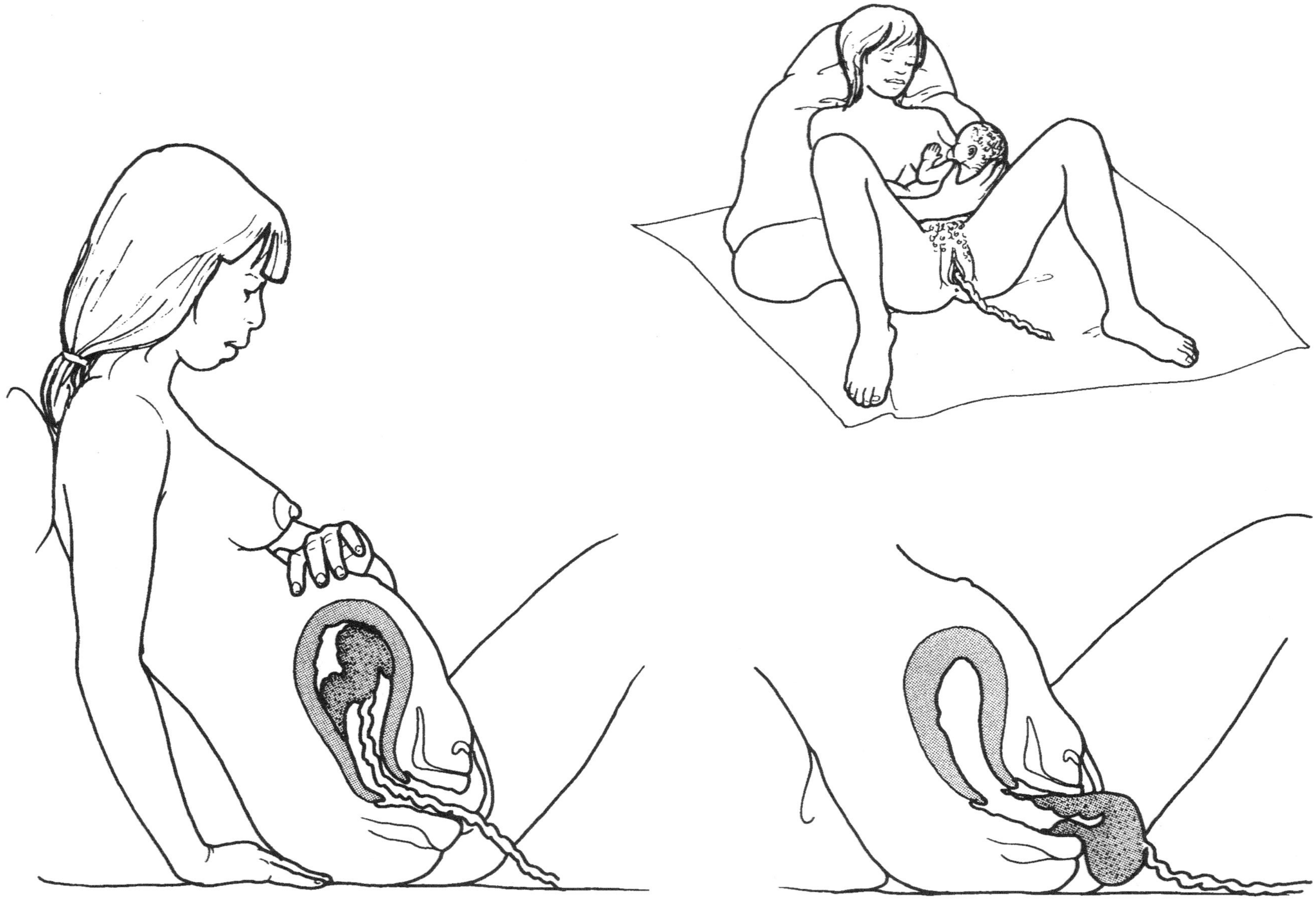

30. Afterbirth — expulsion of the placenta
Soon after the baby is born, the uterus pushes out the placenta. If it does not come out on its own, the abdomen may be lightly massaged to help it come out. If bleeding is heavy or continues, you need medical help.

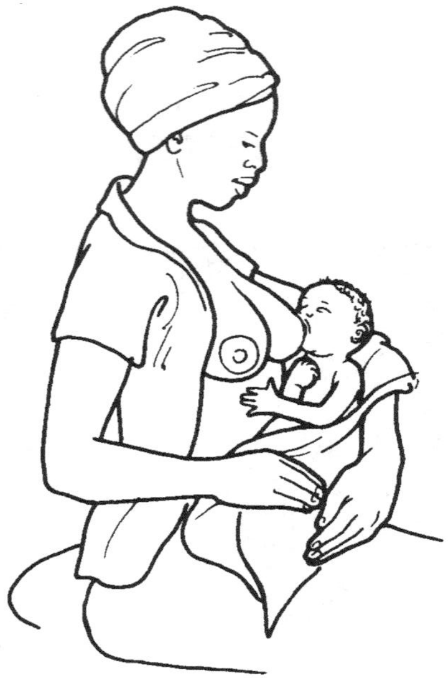

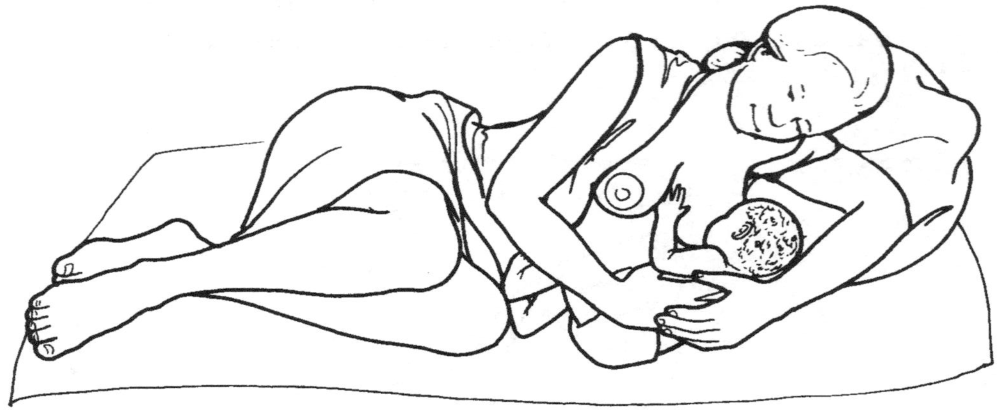

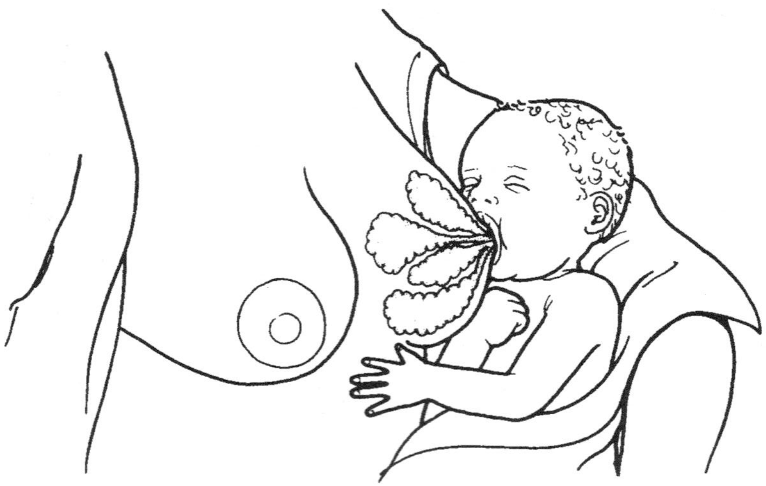

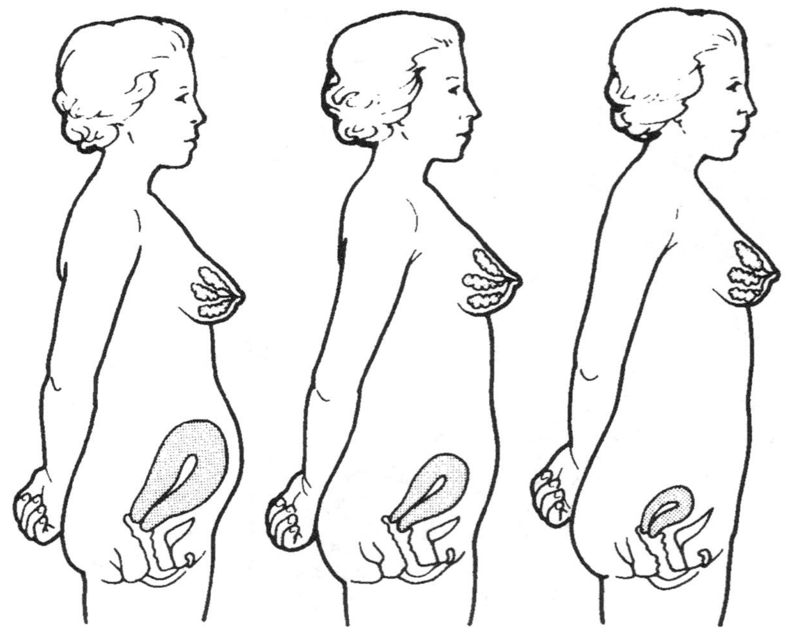

31. Breastfeeding your baby

A newborn baby knows how to suck and should be breastfed within the first hour of life, and then as often as it wants – at least 8-12 times in 24 hours. This helps the milk production and helps the uterus return to normal size.

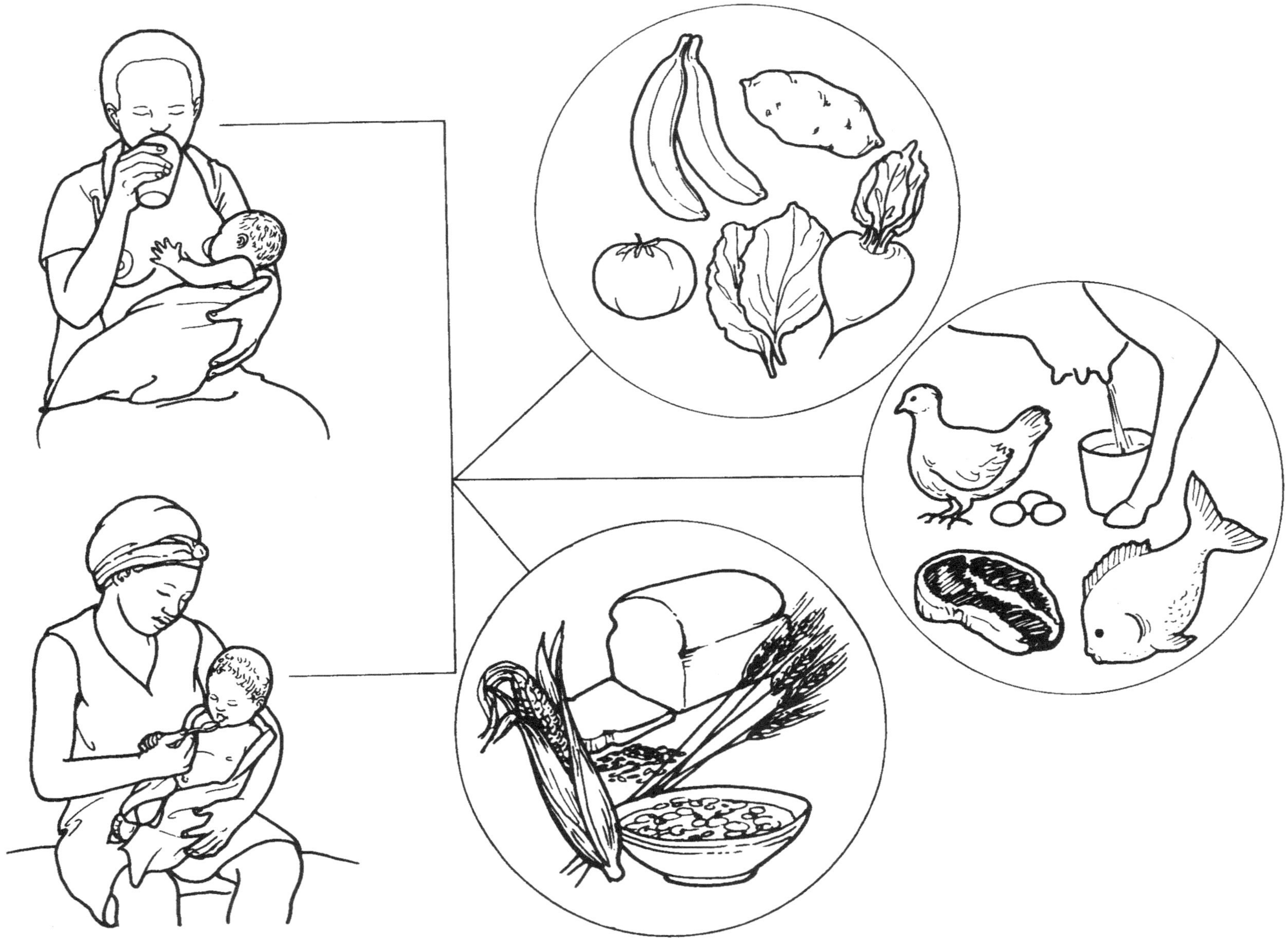

32. Feeding mother and baby

Mother and baby need special care, rest and plenty of good food and fluids. Babies need only breast milk for the first 6 months of life. Breast milk is the best food for the baby. Other liquids are not needed and are not as safe as breast milk.

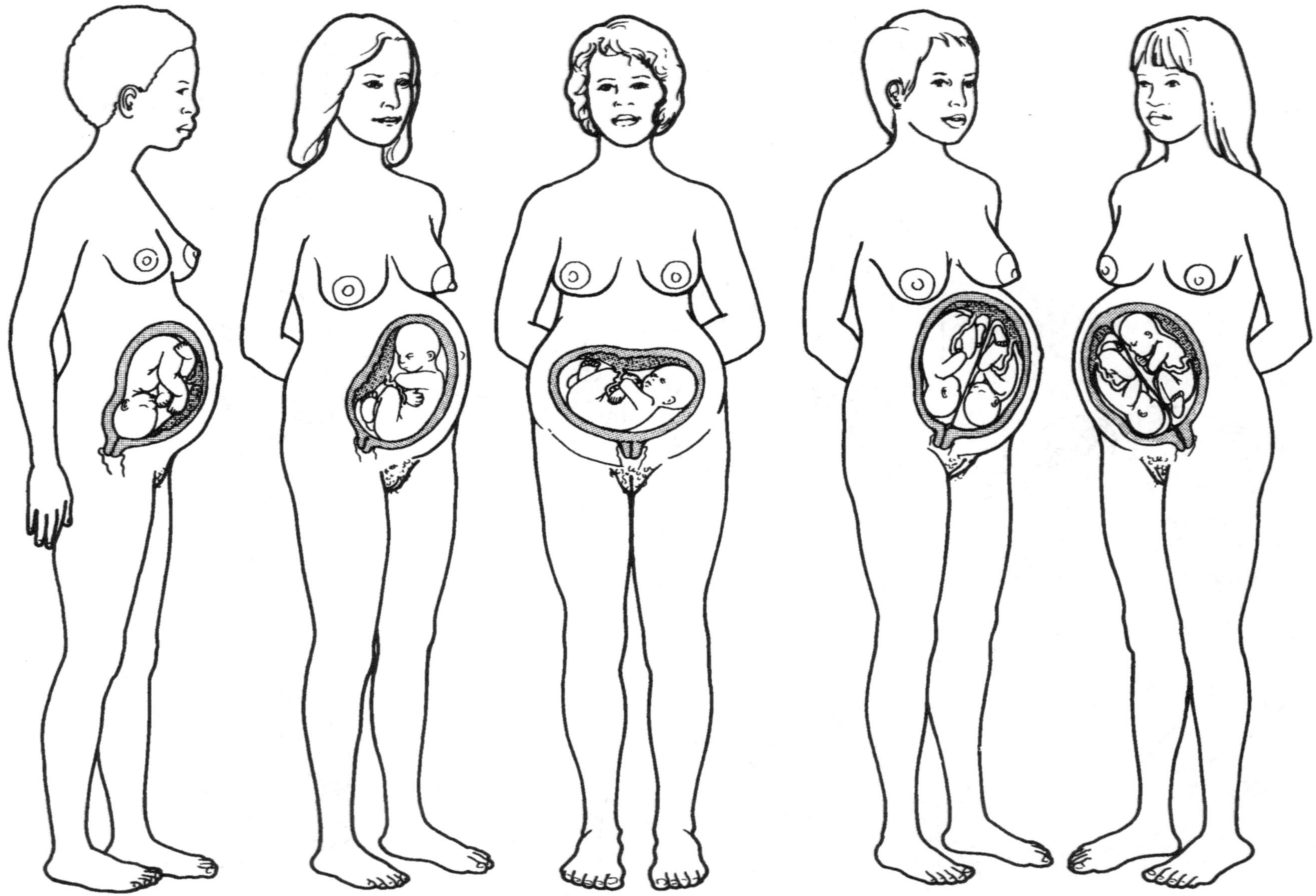

33. Unusual positions of the baby and multiple births

Most babies are born head down, but other positions sometimes happen. Two babies (twins) may sometimes develop, and in rare cases, even more. For these situations, you should get help at a clinic.

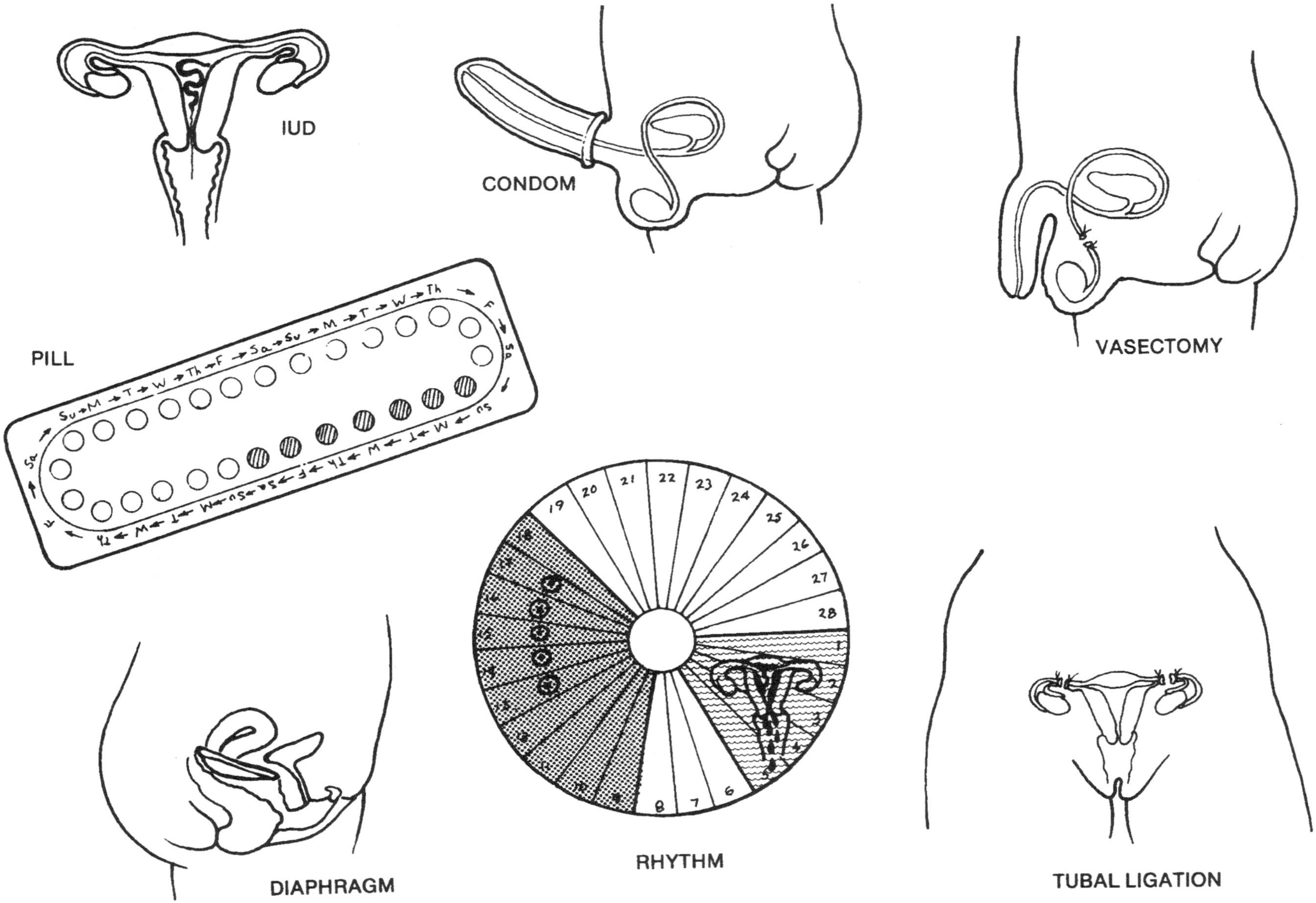

34. Family planning and contraceptives

After we have a baby, our body needs rest, and the baby needs our care. There are many ways to protect ourselves from getting pregnant again.

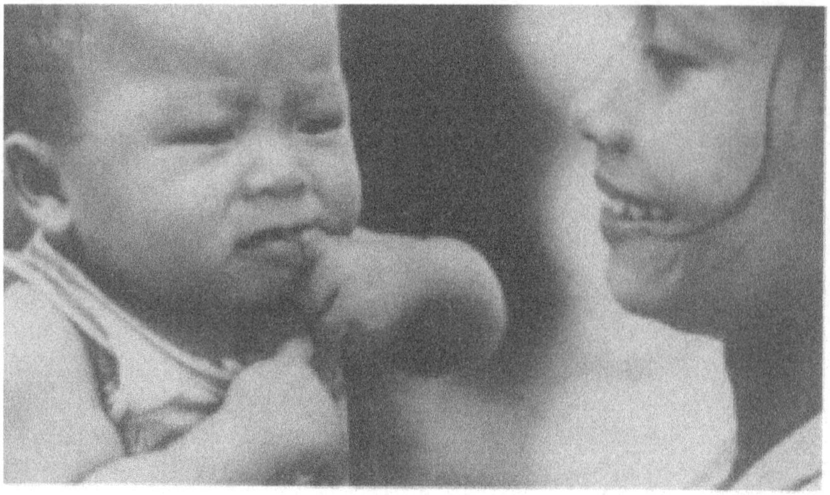
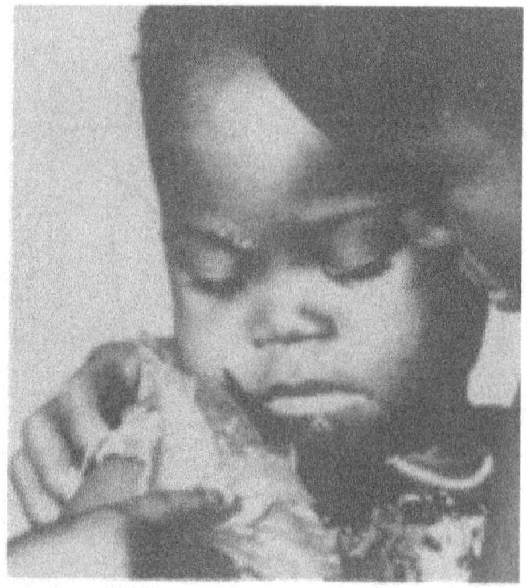
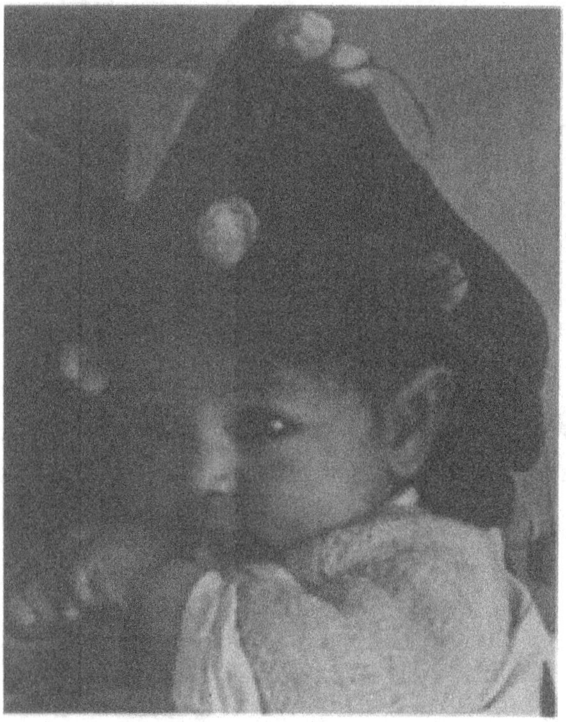
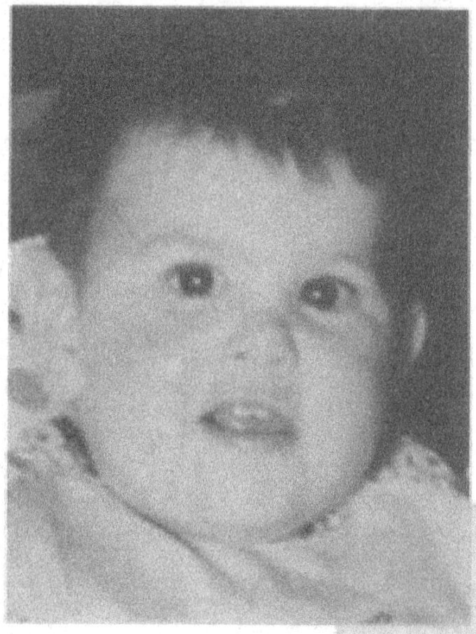
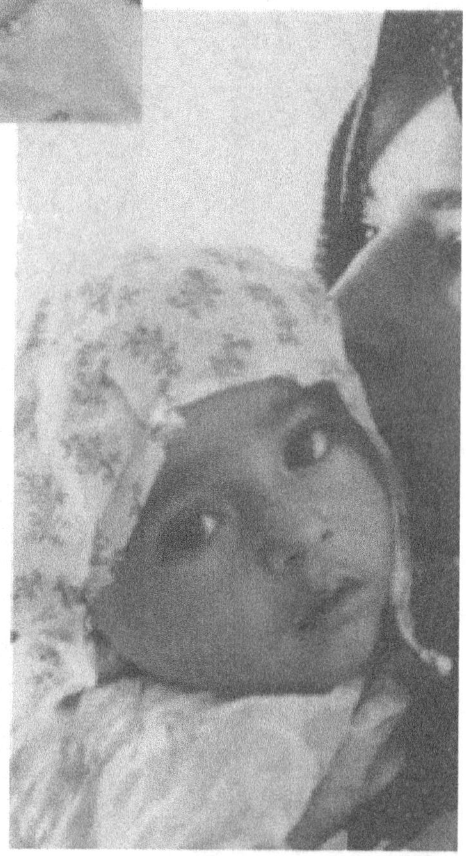
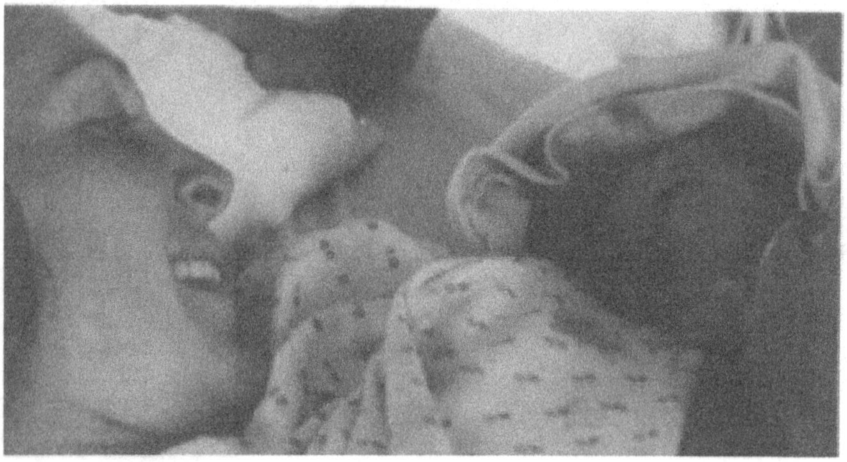

THE CHILDBIRTH PICTURE BOOK

The number of each section here matches the picture with the same number.

1. The female body: Growing from child to woman

To grow from child to woman takes many years. To have healthy children we must wait until our own bodies are fully-grown and strong enough to carry a child, or we may damage ourselves or lose the baby. The ages of the girls in the picture are, starting on the left: 7-9, 10-12, 13-15, and 16-18 years. Change due to puberty (when the reproductive organs become active) begins about the age of 11. Pubic hair begins to grow, the breasts and nipples enlarge — usually after age 11. The pelvis (hips) begins to widen. This process continues until maturity, and full body height and weight are reached at about age 18. There are many variations from this pattern within the normal range of growth. They may be due to individual differences, or to climate and ethnic variations, as well as eating habits and nutrition.

Even if our bodies are physically ready and able to bear a child, we may not be ready in other ways for the responsibilities, the strains and permanent obligations that childbearing and taking care of a child mean.

2. How the female body changes: The breasts and genital organs

We can see changes in our growing bodies in many areas. Our breasts enlarge, as they grow the milk glands that produce milk when we have a baby. The glands are connected by tubes to the nipple, and when we breastfeed, milk comes out of many tiny holes in each nipple.

Our hips widen gradually so we can carry and deliver a baby. Hair begins to grow under the arms and around our genital organs. The hair of the genital area covers and protects the outside of the skinfolds. These skinfolds, called labia (lips) cover the urinary opening and the opening of the vagina. These openings are located in front of the anus.

Because the vagina is close to the anus, and the skin in the genital area is very sensitive, it is important to keep the genital area clean with water and mild soap.

The external body changes we can see are the results of internal changes. This process of change or growing up is called puberty. One sign of puberty — or becoming ready for childbearing — is the start of menstruation (see Picture 4).

3. The internal (inner) female reproductive organs

The internal reproductive organs made for childbearing are the vagina, the uterus (womb), the 2 ovaries, and the 2 Fallopian tubes.

The vagina is the passageway to the uterus. Through this, the sperm (male seeds) enter the uterus during sexual intercourse. At birth, the baby is pushed out through this passage and the external skinfolds, which are elastic and can stretch.

The uterus (womb) is a hollow, oblong (pear shaped) muscle. It has a small opening to the vagina, called the mouth of the uterus (cervix). Inside the uterus, a fertilized egg develops for 9 months until it becomes a baby ready to live outside.

The 2 ovaries contain the egg cells. We are born with all our egg cells, many more than ripen. They become ripe and are released from each ovary, one by one, after we reach puberty. The ovaries are on each side of the uterus. About once a month, an egg cell ripens in one of the ovaries. The ripe egg cell comes out of the ovary (ovulation) and is picked up by the open end of the Fallopian tube next to it. It glides down the Fallopian tube into the hollow uterus. The 2 Fallopian tubes connect the ovaries with the uterus. A ripe egg cell takes several days to travel from the ovary to the uterus; this happens once a month, in between menstruations, and is our most fertile time — the time when we can become pregnant.

4. Menstruation

Menstruation is the monthly discharge of the lining of the uterus. This soft lining, full of small blood vessels, is discharged from our bodies through the vagina; this takes about 4-5 days.

Menstruation happens when a ripe egg cell from one of the ovaries is not fertilized. Our body gets rid of the unfertilized egg cell along with the inner lining of the uterus: this is why we menstruate. The lining of the uterus is renewed each month to make it ready to receive a growing egg if the egg has been fertilized. Menstruation stops usually at age 45 or later.

This monthly bleeding, sometimes called our "period", does us no harm. Sometimes when you have your period you may get cramps, tiredness, and/or a backache. If you are healthy, there is nothing to worry about and you can follow your usual activities: most women do. For instance, women athletes compete regardless of menstruation with no ill effects. It is especially important to wash during menstruation and keep ourselves clean to avoid chafing, soreness and odors.

To absorb the menstrual flow, different kinds of cotton pads or napkins can be used: they should be carefully washed and dried in the sun after use. Also, you can buy disposable sanitary napkins or tampons that are inserted in the vagina. You should investigate to find out which type of sanitary product is most comfortable for you.

5. The external (outer) female reproductive organs

The external genital organs of our bodies, the vulva, consist of double skinfolds that protect the internal organs and the clitoris. The double skinfolds of the labia (or lips) are the outer lips (or big lips — labia majora) and the inner lips (or small lips — labia minora). Like the inside of our mouth, the inside of the skinfolds are moist so that the two sides don't rub against each other and become sore. They cover and protect the opening of the vagina, and the urinary opening just in front of the vagina. This urinary opening is controlled by a strong muscle which holds the tube to the bladder, where urine collects, closed. When the bladder is full, the pressure creates an urge to urinate; during urination (passing water) the muscle relaxes and urine comes out in a stream. Urine should not be held back because it may lead to infection.

The clitoris is located where the labia join in front, forming a hood of skin over this bud-shaped organ. The external genital organs are full of nerve endings and very sensitive to touch. The clitoris, which is an all-important nerve center, is especially sensitive. Stimulation, that is rubbing and touching of the clitoris, results in orgasm (sexual climax), which provides great pleasure and release from tension. Masturbation, which means self-stimulation, is pleasurable and is not harmful, contrary to what is often said.

The clitoris is like the penis of the male, which is also sensitive. Like the penis, the clitoris swells and enlarges due to sexual excitement. It is the source of female orgasm (sexual climax).

A pad of fatty tissue covers the pubic bone in front of the skinfolds of the labia. It is called the "mons Veneris" or the Mount of Venus. This area becomes covered with hair, starting with puberty, and so do the outer surfaces of the labia majora (big lips).

6. The external female reproductive organs

The opening of the vagina is elastic and stretches during sexual intercourse, and in childbirth. A thin piece of skin or membrane called the "hymen" partially covers the opening to the vagina in some women (but not all). This skin is sometimes torn during the first intercourse, which may produce slight bleeding. Often the skin or hymen stretches without tearing or bleeding.

The menstrual flow comes out of the vaginal opening. The triangular area between the vagina and the anus is called the perineum, which has muscles and elastic tissue that stretch greatly during childbirth.

The external genital organs and skinfolds must be carefully handled as any damage in the genital area is extremely painful. In case of injury, strong bleeding may result because there are many blood vessels throughout the genital area.

7. Body changes of pregnancy

Many changes take place in our bodies when we get pregnant and during the 9 months we carry a baby.

The empty uterus is a hollow, pear shaped muscle which takes very little space, located in the middle of our abdomen or pelvis. When it contains a growing baby, the uterus stretches more and more until our abdomen becomes very large. In the last months before the baby is born, the fetus (the baby before birth) fills most of the abdomen. The stretching uterus presses on other internal organs, including the bladder; therefore, we need to urinate more frequently.

Our breasts and nipples also get bigger and ready to provide milk for the baby when it is born. The area around the nipple (the areola) may get darker. Some colostrum, the very first milk, may leak from the nipples before birth, and this is normal.

The position of most babies inside the uterus just before birth is with the head pointed down (Picture 7); a few babies are born in other positions (Picture 33).

8. Body changes of pregnancy

Our bodies change on the outside as well as on the inside, and need special care, good food, and rest during pregnancy. It takes about 9 months for one fertilized egg cell to become a full-grown baby, able to live outside our bodies. The fetus depends entirely on us until it is born. The placenta, which develops early in pregnancy, supplies the fetus with all it needs — in turn, our bodies supply the placenta.

Normally, our weight will increase about 25–35 pounds (11–17 kg); it depends on our usual weight, size and height. To make a healthy baby, we need to not only eat more food, but also a mixed diet of all different kinds of food. (The Food We Need, Picture 17)

9. The male body and reproductive organs

The man's reproductive organs are the testicles and the penis.

The testicles are 2 ball-shaped glands, located in a protective sac called the scrotum. The testicles make the sperm cells (seeds) that fertilize the egg cells made by a woman.

The penis is a tube-shaped organ — located just above and between the 2 testicles; it is usually soft and hangs down. The penis contains a hollow duct that is connected with the bladder, to eliminate urine. The penis is also used to carry the sperm cells, through this same duct, into the vagina. Many millions of these tiny seeds — they are much too small to see — are discharged through the penis in a milky liquid called semen.

10. The male body and reproductive organs

The male body begins to produce sperm cells inside the testicles after reaching puberty, and sperm cells are made for the rest of a man's life. At the same time, pubic hair begins to grow and the muscles of the boy develop. From puberty on, the testicles continuously produce millions of sperm cells. The sperm cells are contained in a milky, white liquid called semen. Each tiny sperm cell has a long tail that propels the cell like a tiny fish.

The tip of the penis, called the glans, is very sensitive to touch as it is full of nerve endings. Touching or lightly rubbing it feels good and causes sexual excitement, much as touching or rubbing the clitoris does. As a result of sexual excitement, and during sexual intercourse, the penis becomes hard, increases in size, and stands up. This is called an erection. A special mechanism pushes the semen from the testicles into the duct of the penis — the same duct that is used to eliminate urine. Then, the semen with the sperm is squirted out, or ejaculated. After ejaculation, the penis shrinks and again becomes limp. Semen may also come out during sleep – this is normal. The sperm cells are so small that more than 500 million are discharged during one ejaculation. Only one sperm cell is needed for each fertilization. Most sperm cells are not used.

The sperm cell of a man determines if a fertilized egg cell develops into a girl or a boy. The sex of the future baby is determined at the moment the sperm cell enters the egg cell (conception).

11. Fertilization

After we reach puberty, each month one egg cell matures in one of our ovaries and is released ("ovulation"). One month the left ovary releases a mature egg cell, the next month, the right ovary does, and so on. We are usually fertile for many years. Menstruation stops some time after age 45. This is called "menopause" and means that we can no longer become pregnant.

About 2 weeks after the beginning our menstrual period a ripe egg cell is released from one of our ovaries. It travels through the Fallopian tube to the uterus; if you have sex 2 weeks after the start of your period, you have the best chance of getting pregnant.

To accomplish fertilization, a sperm cell must meet an egg cell inside our body. Therefore, a man must put his penis inside the vagina and ejaculate. To be able to enter the vagina, the penis first must become hard and erect. This happens due to sexual excitement. At the height of excitement and during orgasm, the semen—the milky fluid full of millions of sperm cells—is pushed out of the penis into the vagina. Many different positions make it possible for the penis to penetrate the vagina. Sperm cells can also enter the vagina if they are ejaculated near its opening, and you can become pregnant even without penetration.

The millions of tiny sperm cells swim around in the vagina after intercourse. Some sperm cells also swim into the uterus through its opening called the cervix, and on into the Fallopian tubes: they may stay alive for up to 3 days inside our bodies.

If a sperm cell meets a ripe egg cell in the Fallopian tube, it may push itself into the much larger egg cell, propelled by its tail. This is called "impregnation". Once the egg cell has been fertilized, no other sperm cell can enter it. The fertilized egg cell — an egg cell which has absorbed a sperm cell — begins to divide and grow.

12. Fertilization

The egg cell, after fertilization by one sperm cell, immediately begins to divide and grow. The fertilized egg cell then continues on its way to the uterus. There it is attached or "implanted" into the soft lining of the uterus, which is filled with tiny blood vessels. If conditions in our body are favorable, it continues to grow in the uterus for 9 months. Each fetus starts with one egg cell and one sperm cell, except in case of some multiple births.

13. Fertilization and beginning of cell division

A ripe egg cell, after leaving the ovary, enters the Fallopian tube and moves towards the uterus. If you recently had sex, the egg cell may meet some sperm cells. The egg is many times bigger than the tiny sperm cells with their long tails that enable them to move rapidly. The sperm cells try to enter the egg, by pushing through the outer cell cover and towards the nucleus or center of the egg cell.

After one sperm cell pushes through the outer covering of the egg cell, the covering becomes hard and no other sperm cell can enter it. Now, the egg cell is fertilized: that means, its center absorbs and combines with the tiny sperm cell. Both together begin to divide over and over, first into 2, then 4, 8, 16 cells and so on. The egg cell starts to divide as soon as it is fertilized and continues on its journey to the uterus. The time from ovulation to fertilization is usually 24-48 hours.

If conditions for growth are good inside the uterus, and if the egg cell and sperm cell are healthy, this may be the beginning of a baby. However, for this tiny clump of cells to become a healthy baby, many other things are also needed: good nourishment and care, as well as sufficient rest for the mother, are most important.

14. Implantation and beginning of growth

When the fertilized and growing egg cell reaches the uterus, it becomes attached to the soft lining of the uterus. That is called "implantation". It happens about 6 days after fertilization. The lining of the uterus, which is full of tiny blood vessels, is now needed for the growth of the fertilized egg. As a result, it is not discharged each month, and menstruation stops. Lack of menstruation ("missing a period") is usually the first sign of pregnancy.

The continuously dividing cluster of cells is implanted in the uterine lining, much like a seed in the ground. The tiny clump of cells grows implanted in the lining of the uterus, from which it gets food, oxygen, and shelter. It takes many weeks before this tiny growth can be seen without a microscope. (Picture 17)

15. Development of the embryo: The first 3 months

Inside the uterus, the clump of cells grows, attached to the soft lining of the uterus, from which it takes its nourishment. This growth is called an "embryo" for the first 3 months. The embryo grows inside protective bag, called the amniotic sac, which develops from the cover of the original egg cell. It is filled with liquid, the amniotic fluid. At 9 weeks, the embryo is still so tiny that it covers only a small part of the palm of a hand, and does not even fill the uterus. (Picture 15)

Inside the protective sac, the head and spine develop first. The embryo still only weighs about 31/2 ounces (96 grams) at the end of 3 months. Ears, eyes and nose can be noticed at 4 months.

16. Development of the embryo: The first 3 months

The placenta is fully developed by about month 3. It is the main source of nourishment for the unborn baby throughout pregnancy. The umbilical cord connects the stomach of the embryo with the placenta. Through the umbilical cord — a thick string of skin containing 2 arteries and a vein – the embryo gets from the placenta what it needs to grow. In turn, the placenta is supplied by the mother. The cord is the baby's lifeline. All nourishment and oxygen, as well as all waste products, pass through the umbilical cord.

During pregnancy, normal exercise is good for you unless you have special problems. You need more rest and sleep when pregnant. During the first few months, you may feel especially tired. Besides more sleep, you need a balanced diet and nourishing food: the first 3 months lay the foundation for a healthy baby. (See "The Food We Need"). A few women get sick to their stomachs during the early months of pregnancy. If vomiting is severe you should seek medical help.

A miscarriage – which means that the content of the uterus comes out unexpectedly – happens most often during the first 3 months of pregnancy if there is something wrong with the embryo, or it cannot grow. The first 3 months are also the safest time for abortion. After a miscarriage, any remaining growth must be cleaned out of the uterus, or an infection may start. You should visit a clinic or doctor and have an examination. Having a miscarriage does not mean you cannot get pregnant or have a healthy baby. After your period comes back, you can still get pregnant and have a successful pregnancy and healthy baby.

17. The food we need

To have a healthy baby, we must keep healthy and take good care of ourselves. It is important to eat enough, as well as eating the right kinds of foods, since we have to feed a growing baby who depends on what we eat. When we are pregnant, we need more food and a variety of different foods and plenty of liquids.

We should eat a mixed diet that includes foods from all the basic food groups (Picture 17). Protein containing foods, such as meat, fish, eggs, cheese and beans are important. We also need different kinds of cereals and grains, such as rice, corn, wheat and whole grain breads. Fresh vegetables, including leafy ones, and fresh fruit, such as bananas, oranges, apples and berries are good for you and your developing baby. Potatoes, carrots, and other root vegetables should be part of what you eat regularly. To assure enough iron and vitamins, many women take vitamins with iron tablets during pregnancy. Such tablets can supplement a good diet, but not replace it.

18. What to avoid

Your baby's growth and health depends on what you eat and drink. What you put in your body is passed on to the fetus through the placenta.

Alcohol taken regularly or in large amounts is not good for you, and it is especially bad for the growing fetus. Smoking is a health hazard for everyone: it is especially hazardous to your baby's health and you should stop smoking, especially during your pregnancy. Coffee and other stimulants, if taken in large amounts, not only may trouble you, but they are even more troublesome for your unborn baby.

If you need to take medicine or prescription drugs for any health problems, you should tell the physician or clinic who prescribed the drug you are pregnant. Some medicines can harm your unborn baby and may need to be changed.

19. Familiar foods we know and eat

To the teacher or group leader: Please prepare a short text on locally available foods and paste that text onto the blank picture page.

What combinations of locally available foods constitute a "balanced diet" as outlined in the text and Picture 17? Please also see suggestions provided for Picture 19, the text should be coordinated with this picture. Outline the preparation of the most frequently eaten local foods/dishes, and discuss their food values. Depending on where you teach/live, a discussion on growing/planting some of the nourishing local foods may be included, as may costs of foods/dishes, time of preparation and where/how to shop for best foods.

The aim is to show with examples of locally available foods, how to arrive at a balanced diet that includes all-important food values at lowest cost, on a regular basis (every day).

20. The development of the pregnancy

The development and growth of the fetus takes about 9 months inside the uterus. During the first half of the pregnancy, the changes of our body are hardly visible – most of them take place on the inside. The first noticeable change is that menstruation stops. If menstruation is 2 or more weeks late, you can have a test at a local hospital or clinic to know for sure if you are pregnant. If you cannot go through with the pregnancy, the safest time for abortion is as early as possible, or before 3 months.

During the last 3 months, the abdomen becomes larger very quickly because the fetus puts on a lot of weight. In Picture 20, the first 6 months of pregnancy are shown in the top row of figures; the last 3 months are shown in the bottom row. The last picture shows the final stage of pregnancy; the fetus has dropped in the uterus and is about to be born.

Regular prenatal care is important for you to monitor the development of the baby and to prevent any unexpected problems in delivery.

21. The development of the pregnancy

The embryo develops inside the amniotic sac (bag of waters), and can move about freely, protected by the amniotic fluid, which acts as a cushion and maintains a constant temperature. After the embryo has been growing for more than 12 weeks (that means you have missed your period 3 times) it is still very small. Only after 4 months or so do you begin to "show". The breasts also enlarge and the areola, the dark area around the nipples, may grow wider and darker.

The embryo is called a fetus after all the major organ systems have begun to develop. At about 20 weeks, you may begin to feel movement. At first, the movement of the fetus can be hardly felt; later, it becomes stronger and we can feel the fetus kick.

The sex of the baby to be born is determined at fertilization by the male sperm cell. The embryo for the first 8 weeks looks the same, whether male or female: after 8 weeks, distinctive female/male sexual organs begin to form.

22. The development of the pregnancy

By the end of pregnancy, you may find it difficult to bend down or move quickly. The whole body feels heavy and out of balance. You may also have to urinate more because the fetus is very large and presses on the bladder. It also presses on the lungs so you may be short of breath.

To determine the probable day of the baby's birth, count back 3 months from the first day of your last menstrual cycle and add one year and 7 days. For example, if your last menstruation started January 8, you may expect to deliver about the middle of October. The duration of pregnancy is about 280 days or 40 weeks from the date of your last menstrual period, but anything between 37 weeks and up to 42 weeks is normal. If you feel labor pains before 37 weeks, or if you pregnancy is continuing after 42 weeks, you should get medical help quickly.

23. Just before birth

By 9 months, the fetus weighs about 7-8 lb (3-4 kg.). Some newborn babies weigh as much as 11 lb (5 kg.). The one cell at fertilization has become 200 billion cells when the baby is ready to be born.

During the last month before birth, the fetus is fully developed, puts on more weight, and develops a layer of fat. In Picture 23, you can see the umbilical cord connected to the placenta and how the fetus fits into the very small space, filling most of the uterus with very little room to move. The cervix, the opening from the uterus to the vagina, is still completely closed. The position of the fetus shown here, with the head down, is the usual one for birth. Earlier, the fetus may have been head-up, or in many different positions. The head down position is the best for delivery for both mother and baby. Deliveries with the baby in other positions may need special help and should be done in the hospital.

Your body knows when the baby is ready to be born, and can live outside the uterus. The baby remains attached to the umbilical cord until after the birth. Only when the baby is outside the womb and can breathe for itself, is the cord no longer needed.

24. The beginning of labor

Before the baby is born, it moves down inside the uterus, head first, against the cervix. Sometimes, the bag or sac, which contains the fetus and the fluid in which it has grown for 9 months, breaks first, and fluid comes out of the vagina (when this happens, we say that the "water breaks"). Soon afterwards, labor pains, strong radiating pains in the back, lower belly, or both, begin. Sometimes, labor pains start before the "water breaks". The onset of labor is different for each woman and each pregnancy.

What causes labor pains? The uterus is a strong muscle which holds the baby; it contracts to push the baby out. When it is time for the baby to be born, the mouth of the uterus must open up to let the baby out. This is the first stage of labor. The contractions of the uterus are involuntary; that means we cannot control, start, or stop them. They start on their own when your baby is ready. Sometimes labor is "induced" (started artificially), but unless there is a problem it is best to wait for labor to begin naturally.

At first, the contractions that open up the cervix and push the baby into the birth canal are far apart; perhaps every half-hour. They become more frequent until they are only 2 minutes apart, and may cause great pain.

25. The birth process

You can help yourself and help the baby be born by breathing deeply and slowly during contractions. This helps your muscles relax. If you know what is happening, you need not be afraid. Being afraid makes your body tense. There are also drugs against pain that are safe to use. Discuss this with the person (midwife/ physician) who will attend your delivery to find out what is available where you live and what drugs are safe for you and your baby.

Childbirth classes for parents-to-be teach special exercises and breathing patterns in preparation for a safe delivery. They explain what is happening to your body during, before, and after birth. If childbirth classes do not exist where you live, you may want to form a group and find a teacher, and/or get institutional support to get them organized.

The birth position shown in Picture 25 and in the following ones, is with the mother's back propped up to enable her to push the baby down — with the weight of the baby helping the delivery. It is a comfortable position for most women that can be arranged on a bed, or a specially cleaned and prepared area on a mat or on the floor.

During the first stage of labor, the uterus pushes the baby down against the cervix (mouth of the womb). With each contraction, this opening gets bigger until the cervix is fully open or dilated, to let the baby out. This sometimes takes many hours of labor. With the first baby, it may take an 12-14 hours or more. With the second and following births, it usually takes a much shorter time.

During the second stage of labor, the working stage, the baby is pushed into the birth canal and then the external genitalia, the vulva, begin to stretch. By pushing and bearing down with each contraction, we can help during this second stage of labor with the birth of the baby.

26. The birth process

The same birth process shown in Picture 25 is shown in Picture 26, seen from outside. The head of the baby turns while it is pushed out, which makes it easier, especially since it has to come through the tight opening of the vagina. The outer skin has to stretch a great deal to let the baby through. This is called "crowning". The baby turns as it comes through the birth canal, and is pushed out through the elastic skin-folds of the vulva as shown in Picture 26.

The bones of the baby's head are not completely hard, but can mold with the narrow passage it must go through. Once the head is out, the shoulders and the rest of the body follow very quickly through the slippery, soft tissues of the vulva.

The perineum – the skin and muscles surrounding the opening between the vagina and the anus – must be elastic and give with each push. If this outer skin cannot stretch enough it may tear — this is painful and must be closed with stitches. To avoid perineal tears, you should not push too much during crowning. A cut, called an "episiotomy", is sometimes made in the perineum to let the baby's head out more quickly. However, such a cut has to be stitched again and that may make problems with future deliveries. It may be better to take more time to let the baby's head out more slowly. In a well-managed, normal delivery, neither an episiotomy nor tearing should happen unless the baby is very big. The average weight of a newborn is about 7 lb (3.18 kg.) and the average length about 20 inches (50.8 cm.). There are many variants from this average, depending on the parents, the ethnic group, and whether the baby is born early or late, environmental factors, health and nutrition of the mother, and more.

27. Birth positions of mothers

Women around the world give birth in different positions (Picture 27). Between contractions, you may stand up, walk around, drink nourishing liquids and light solids, and talk with the midwife, your husband/partner, or mother, who have come to encourage and support you during labor. Many hospitals encourage the father-to-be, relatives, or friends to stay with a birthing woman at a time when each woman most depends on help. You should find a midwife or doctor and hospital who provide what you want, and make arrangements ahead of time.

It is easy to see that if you sit or lie with your back propped up, or are on hands and knees, the weight of the baby helps the contractions of the uterus to push the baby out. To lie flat on your back with the legs up makes labor more difficult and painful; because in that position, our bodies must push the baby up, instead of down.

Labor is hard work — the hardest and most strenuous work there is. During the hours of labor, a mother-to-be needs personal attention, support and care.

28. Birth

The skinfolds and muscles of the vulva will stretch to let the baby's head out gradually. A trained nurse/midwife should help you throughout the labor and delivery. A doctor should be available in case any problems arise. Your husband/partner, mother, or a friend can be very supportive.

Most babies are born head first. The normal birth process takes time and encouragement of the mother in her hard work: there should be no interference or pulling of the baby. An episiotomy or cut in the perineum to let the baby's head out should not be done unless really necessary.

The baby starts breathing and crying right away. The mucus must be removed from its nose and mouth immediately. If the baby does not breathe, mouth-to-mouth resuscitation must be started at once, or the baby may die or be permanently brain damaged for lack of oxygen.

At birth, the baby is wet, and often covered with a white, greasy substance called "vernix" which does not need to be removed. The baby, as soon as it comes out, should be given to the mother to hold, or placed on her abdomen or chest, where it will be warm and safe.

Birth is a difficult experience for the baby, who is pushed hard through some very narrow spaces. It also means that the baby must adjust immediately to a quite new environment: its very life depends on it! The newborn should be handled gently, and with loving care.

29. Immediate newborn care

The baby should begin to breathe and cry at once. Both nose and mouth must be cleared of mucus immediately; if the baby does not breathe, mouth-to-mouth resuscitation must be started immediately.

The baby should placed skin to skin on the mother's abdomen or chest. The baby is usually alert and awake, and should breastfeed within the first hour of life. The first milk, colostrum, is the healthiest liquid the baby could ever eat. If baby and mother are healthy, there is no need to separate them to do routine hospital tests, or to put the baby underneath warming lights. The mother's chest will keep the baby warm.

The umbilical cord can be cut when the baby is on the mother's chest, when the cord has stopped pulsating and has become much thinner and pale. The cord should be tied in 2 places — one close to the baby. Then, it is cut between the ties with a sterile razor blade or sterile scissors that have been boiled in water for 15 minutes. The stump should be kept dry and clean, and will fall off in a few days.

30. Expulsion of the placenta

After the baby is born, some more contractions push out the afterbirth (placenta). Usually, this happens about 10 minutes after the baby comes out, or even later. The placenta should never be pulled out. By lightly massaging the abdomen, the placenta can be detached. After that, the uterus contracts again tightly and pulls back.

Suckling on the breasts will stimulate contractions to expel the placenta. The infant will gain much needed protection against infection, as well as nutrition, from the first breast milk, "colostrum". Besides, this suckling stimulates milk production. It is important for the mother to feed and hold close her newborn to establish the life-long, loving bonds between mother and child.

Some bleeding during and after the birth is normal. With good care, rest, and nourishing food, the blood we lose will soon be replaced with no harm to our bodies. But, if the bleeding is heavy (more than 2 cups) or does not stop, medical help should be sought at once. After the birth, it is important not to overdo activities, but, it is good to stand up and walk around a little, soon after a normal delivery.

31. Breastfeeding your baby

The first milk, "colostrum" is critically important for the baby's health. Often, right after the birth, both mother and baby are wide awake, and the baby will nurse well at the breast within the first hour of life. This early nursing helps to stimulate the milk supply. The mother and baby may then feel tired, and sleep for 8-10 hours. After that, the baby should eat at the breast 8-12 times in 24 hours. In some cultures, the baby is worn against the breast and feeds more frequently than that. The more a baby nurses, the more milk our breasts produce. Breast milk is the most nourishing food for a baby and contains many important antibodies that protect the baby against all kinds of disease. Breastfeeding also helps the uterus to contract and go back to normal size.

Breastfeeding should not hurt. It is important that the baby "latch on" well by attaching to the breast with a wide open mouth, so that the pressure when the baby sucks is on the breast and not the nipple. If breastfeeding is very painful, take the baby off the breast, and reattach, making sure that the mouth is wide open when the baby attaches. If you stroke the baby's cheek with your nipple, the baby will open his mouth and "root" for the nipple.

You will make only a few spoonfuls of milk at first, but this is enough for the baby. About 3 days after the birth, your breasts will start to feel more full and a lot more milk will be made. All babies lose weight in the first few days, but they should regain their birthweight by 2 weeks of life. Over the first few days, the baby should stool (poop) 2-3 times a day, and the stool should change from black and sticky to yellow and liquid. Liquid poop is normal in a breastfed baby and is not a sign of diarrhea.

The World Health Organization states that no other fluids besides breast milk are needed until the baby is 6 months old. As long as the baby has access to the breast, you do not need to give water, teas, solids, or other milks for 6 months.

There are health risks associated with feeding the baby anything else besides breast milk in the first 6 months. Infant formula is the safest alternative to breast milk as it is more nutritionally complete than animal milk. But infant formula does not protect against infection, and in countries where clean water, refrigeration, and sterilization are not available, any kind of non-breast milk feeding carries a high risk of making the baby very sick. Infants who do not get breast milk are more likely to die in the first year of life than infants who are breastfed.

32. Feeding mother and baby

You do not need a special diet to produce good milk, though you need to eat some extra food and drink plenty of fluid, as you are feeding yourself and the baby! We should eat regularly from the basic food groups (Picture 32): meat, fish and dairy products, and beans for protein; cereals and grains, bread, rice, corn, vegetables and fruit. You will often feel thirsty when breastfeeding. Drink extra fluids – but you do not need to drink milk to make milk! (Cows, goats, and other milk-making mammals do not drink milk to make milk!).

33. Unusual positions of the baby and multiple births

Not all babies are born head first. The positions in Picture 33 are unusual, with the baby lying across (transverse), the most difficult to deliver. A "breech birth" means the baby is born feet first. If the feet come out and it takes a long time for the head to be born, the baby may not get enough oxygen, which may cause brain damage. All unusual positions make birth more difficult and dangerous for mother and baby. In these cases you may need a cesarean section, where the baby is born through a cut in the abdominal wall and the uterus. This operation must be done in the hospital with anesthesia.

Identical twins occur if a single egg cell, fertilized by one sperm cell, splits: they share the same placenta. Twins can also develop from 2 separate egg cells, fertilized by different sperm cells; each one has its own placenta, and they may be of different sex and look different.

Twins occur once in about 87 pregnancies. Triplets or quadruplets are much more rare. Like twins, they may be from one egg cell which splits, or they may be from several egg cells which come out of the ovary at the same time and are all fertilized by different sperm cells. Twins and multiple births are usually discovered before delivery because of the large size of the abdomen. But, sometimes, they come as a surprise. In the case of twins or multiple births, special care of the mother is needed.

34. Family planning and contraceptives

After you have a healthy baby, your body needs rest. You and your children will be healthier and stronger if you space your pregnancies. You may also decide to have no more children.

There are many different ways to protect yourself from becoming pregnant again. Different methods of preventing pregnancy are available to women or men and can be used by you or your partner. The "Pill" prevents ovulation; the IUD (Intra Uterine Device) prevents conception or implantation, and has to be put into the uterus by a midwife or doctor. You can put a diaphragm into the vagina yourself before intercourse, it closes off the entrance to the uterus, as does a cervical cap. To get the right size, you need to be measured at a clinic. Foams and jellies that kill sperm can be inserted in the vagina before having sex.

The male contraceptive is the condom. This covers the penis during intercourse and stops sperm from getting into the vagina. It is effective, easy to use, and has no bad effects, and can help to prevent sexually transmitted diseases such as AIDS (HIV).

When you have completed your family, you can permanently prevent fertilization in men and women. Men can have a vasectomy, and an operation called "tubal ligation" (the cutting of the Fallopian tubes) can be performed in women.

It is important to get detailed information about contraceptives. Some may have adverse side effects on your body, and you need to find what is best for you. If not used properly, contraceptives will not prevent pregnancy. Ask at a family planning clinic for more information.

THE CHILDBIRTH PICTURE BOOK

Leader's Guide: Discussion Points

To all group leaders and teachers

These discussion points are based on the pictures of the CBPB and are designed to stimulate group participation. They are, first of all, for training workshops and childbirth classes of all kinds. They also can be used for sex and family planning education, and women's health groups. They are meant to encourage open communication on reproductive health and childbirth.

This Guide can serve women, husbands, fathers-to-be, partners, grandmothers, children, and especially teenagers. Families should be invited to special sessions to establish understanding and family support for the mother-to-be, to make the stressful process of birth into a shared and happy family event. The goal of the book is to reach the widest audiences, regardless of language and literacy: the pictures tell the story — the presentation of the text and the discussion points are based on oral communication; therefore, many important concepts are deliberately repeated and/or presented in different ways, always encouraging questions and discussion.

As leader, you might want to first review the text with the pictures. You may want to make some changes and/or add questions that might be of special interest for your particular group and locality.

The purpose of this book is to explain normal conditions which are shared by almost all women. Unusual situations are not included here, as they need special and professional attention. These discussion points are based on the most frequently asked questions concerning normal childbirth situations and reproductive health, rather than problems and exceptions which are not included in this basic program. Even when problems are mentioned (miscarriage, unusual positions of baby) they are not explained in detail. You may want to discuss "problems" in a follow up after the normal biological information has been absorbed. Other publications should be consulted for further information and special situations.

Local myths and beliefs

The biological facts in this book are often are incompatible with local myths and traditions, many of which are damaging to women (myths about menstruation/food habits and taboos, etc.). The leader will need skill and tact to lead discussions that pay respect to local beliefs, but ensure that participants understand the biological facts for what they are.

For group meetings

It is important that all participants can see the pictures during the discussion. Copies of the books can be distributed if necessary so everyone can see the pictures and participate.
The Discussion Points are grouped according to topic. The outline provided here should be amplified with local information. Birth positions and customs, as well as contraceptive practices need to have local experience and information added.

Discussion points

The following outline provides a framework for your own teaching plan. The succession of information in each picture is from left to right, and from top to bottom.
Start each presentation by going through the entire series of pictures first. Read the text out loud, allowing plenty of time with each picture, pointing to specific figures/details of the picture that is discussed.

For all pictures

Show both pictures on each page together, and read the text underneath. When you have made the discussion points, encourage the group to ask questions and participate.

The female body: Growth and changes — Pictures 1 & 2

Discussion points:

- Growth and development of body takes many years. Talk about ages of figures, (from left to right: 7-9 years, 10-12 years, 13-15 years, 16-18 years). Variations happen due to differences between individuals, ethnic groups, nutrition, climate, etc.
- Development of breasts: As breasts enlarge, important changes take place inside. Point to breasts: in these glands, the milk is made. When the baby sucks on the nipple, the milk flows through the milk ducts to the baby's mouth.
- Development of genitalia: (pointing to genitalia): Genitalia enlarge and become covered with hair-which protects the opening of the vagina and the urinary opening.
- When are you ready for childbearing? The female body must be fully grown (fourth figure on right-picture one) before starting a pregnancy. You should wait until you are ready for the responsibility of child care.
- Early childbearing is dangerous both mother and baby may be harmed by too early childbirth.

Internal reproductive organs and menstruation — Pictures 3 & 4

Discussion points:

- Egg Cell (Ovum): We are born with all our egg cells, but they do not become ripe and are not released until puberty. Though an egg cell is the largest cell of our body, it is visible only with a microscope.
- Timing: After we reach puberty, one ripe egg cell is released every month (about 28 days): the first month from the left ovary, the second month from the right ovary, and so on. (Sometimes the time may be more than 4 weeks).
- Journey of Egg Cell (Picture 4): Show progress of egg cell from upper left picture to lower right, and the discharge. The egg cell, when it is ripe, is picked up or sucked up by the wide, open end of the Fallopian tube near the ovary. The tiny egg cell then slowly slips down the Fallopian tube to the uterus: this journey takes several days.
- Menstruation: When the ripe egg cell reaches the uterus without being fertilized, it is discarded by our body. The inner, blood-filled lining of the uterus also is eliminated through the vagina because it is not needed. This takes several days and is the reason why we bleed every month if we are not pregnant. This is "Menstruation".
- Protection during Menstruation: Different kinds of clean, cotton, or disposable pads can be worn for protection during menstruation. Or, absorbent tampons can be inserted into the vagina. Discuss the sanitary products available locally and how to deal with menstruation.
- Menstrual pains: Usually you can follow all your normal activities. Sometimes, cramps may accompany menstruation. If you have severe pain, and/or any unusual discharge, go to a clinic or seek professional help. Wash the genital area often, and especially during menstruation, to avoid chafing and soreness. Normal washing and bathing during menstruation is good for you.

The external reproductive organs — Pictures 5 & 6
Discussion points:

- Location of external organs: explain front and side views.
- Protection: External organs, the vulva, are the labia minora (small or inner lips) and the labia majora (large or outer lips). These double skinfolds and the pubic hair protect the body openings.
- The opening to the vagina is surrounded by soft skinfolds that are elastic and stretch during sexual intercourse and childbirth. A thin piece of skin called the "hymen" partially closes the vaginal opening of some women, but not all. The hymen either stretches or tears with the first sexual intercourse (penetration). If the hymen is torn, this may result in slight bleeding. If there is no hymen, or if it stretches, there is no bleeding. Each woman is different—the absence of bleeding does not mean that sexual intercourse (penetration) has taken place before.
- The menstrual flow comes out of the vaginal opening.
- The urinary opening (urethral meatus) is just in front of the vaginal opening. It is controlled by a strong muscle which holds the bladder closed. The bladder is where urine is collected.
- Urination (Passing water): When the bladder is full, you feel an urge to urinate. When the voluntary muscles are relaxed, the collected fluid comes out. During the last month of pregnancy, the fetus crowds the belly and presses on the bladder, so you need to urinate more often.
- Retention of urine is dangerous because urine contains many waste products. If urine is held back, the abdomen becomes bloated and painful: go to a hospital or clinic for help at once.
- The function of the clitoris is to make sexual intercourse enjoyable. The clitoris is full of nerve endings and very sensitive to touch. The clitoris is an all-important nerve center and focus of our female sexuality. The clitoris is biologically similar to the male penis: Stimulation (rubbing) of the clitoris results in orgasm (sexual climax). Protection: The clitoris is well protected by the skinfolds of the labia (lips) and by a hood because it is very sensitive and is connected with the nerve centers in our brain.
- The skinfolds over the vaginal opening and the clitoris are full of nerve endings and glands. This is the most sensitive area of our body and easily damaged. The genital area needs to be carefully handled; any damage is very painful and may create serious problems due to infection.
- Cleanliness: Washing and cleanliness of the genital area is important because the elimination of urine and feces (urinary opening and anus) takes place nearby.

Body changes of pregnancy — Pictures 7 & 8
Discussion points:

- The uterus is a hollow, oblong, pear-shaped muscle that can stretch. Normally, it is so small it cannot be felt from outside. At the end of a pregnancy, it fills most of the abdomen, which bulges because of the size of the uterus. Compare empty and pregnant uterus: Show and describe fetus, placenta, cord, etc.
- Breasts: the milk glands develop as the breasts enlarge and get ready for milk production.
- Weight gain: Normally, your weight will increase 3-4 times the weight of the baby, sometimes more.

The male body and reproductive organs; fertilization — Pictures 9-11
Discussion points:

- Growth and development of the male body. At puberty, pubic hair begins to grow, the boy's muscles develop, and the testicles begin to produce sperm cells (male seeds).

- Sperm cell production: the testicles keep producing many millions of sperm cells from the time of puberty throughout a man's life. A sperm cell is much smaller than an egg cell (see Picture 12).
- The penis is a tube-shaped, soft organ which normally is limp and hangs down. It is sensitive to touch, especially at the tip (called glans), which contains many nerve endings, much like the clitoris of the female.
- The urinary opening is in the tip of the penis: the same duct that carries urine also carries the male sperm cells.
- Discharge of sperm cells/Ejaculation: After sperm cell production begins at puberty, extra sperm cells are discharged sometimes, usually during sleep. This is called ejaculation. The sperm cells are so small that more than 500 million are discharged with each ejaculation. They are contained in a milky white substance called semen. Each sperm cell has a tiny head and a long tail that lets it move or swim like a fish.
- Erection: An erection results from sexual excitement. Sexual excitement of a man may result from touching the sensitive part of the penis, like sexual excitement in a woman results from touching the sensitive clitoris. Sexual excitement makes the penis swell, become erect and hard. Then, a special mechanism pushes the semen out of the penis and ejaculation takes place. Then, the penis becomes limp again.
- Sexual Intercourse/Penetration: means that the erect penis is pushed into the vagina and ejaculates due to sexual excitement. The climax of sexual excitement is called orgasm. Millions of tiny sperm cells in the liquid semen are ejaculated into the vagina as a result of male orgasm.
- Orgasm is the sexual climax experienced by both women and men due to sexual excitement, as a result of stimulation (rubbing) of the clitoris or penis, and/or during sexual intercourse.
- Different positions of sexual intercourse: Many different positions can be assumed for penetration (sexual intercourse).
- The journey of the sperm cells (Point out each organ and the journey of the sperm cells): After the sperm cells are deposited in the vagina (contained in the milky fluid of the semen) they swim all over the vagina including into the uterus and on into the Fallopian tubes. Many millions of them swim about for up to 3 days. If they meet a ripe egg cell in one of the Fallopian tubes, one of the tiny sperm cells may enter the much larger egg cell. This is called fertilization (impregnation). The sperm cell has reached the end of its journey.
- Most of the sperm cells contained in the semen come back out of the vagina. It is important to wash the vaginal area and to keep it clean.

Fertilization; implantation; beginning of growth — Pictures 12, 13, 14
Discussion points:

- Fertilization (conception): Picture 12. The egg cell is round with a center (nucleus). It is much bigger than a sperm cell. When a sperm cell meets an egg cell, it tries to push through the outer wall of the egg cell, into the center. If the sperm cell succeeds, the outer wall becomes hard and no other sperm cell can enter. The head of the sperm cell and the center of the egg cell combine and the fertilized egg begins to divide.
- Cell Division: It takes about 30 hours for the fertilized egg cell to divide for the first time. Each cell, in turn, divides over and over until a clump of cells is formed. It takes 4 days for the clump of cells shown in Picture 12 to form (middle of lower row).
- Journey of the fertilized egg cell: The fertilized egg, while dividing, continues its journey through the Fallopian tube to the uterus. (Picture 13).
- Implantation: (Picture 14). When the tiny clump of cells gets to the uterus, it settles into the soft, blood-filled lining. This is called implantation. The lining of the uterus is no longer discarded each month because it is needed: that means menstruation stops.

- Beginning of growth: If all the conditions are good, the tiny clump of cells continues to grow, implanted in the lining of the uterus, from where it draws its nourishment. The cells divide over and over. But it takes many weeks before this growth can even be seen without enlargement by a microscope.
- How do you know you are pregnant? The first sign an egg has been fertilized is that menstruation stops. To be certain, you can do a pregnancy test. (Discuss tests available in your area).

Development of the embryo: The first 3 months — Pictures 15 & 16

Discussion points:

- Formation of embryo: After several weeks of growth, the embryo begins to form inside the cover of the egg cell. This cell cover becomes a protective bag or sac, filled with liquid. It is called the amniotic sac filled with the amniotic fluid. The placenta also begins to develop.
- Time: It takes 3 months before the embryo is big enough to cover a small part of your hand.
- Changes: You cannot see outside changes in the first 3 months, as the embryo is so small. But, you may experience other changes: for instance, some women are sick to their stomachs. Other women are very tired and need a lot of sleep. The breasts and nipples also enlarge.
- The growth of the embryo (Picture 16). One month after fertilization, (drawing on left), to 3 months after fertilization (drawing on right). It takes 3 months for the embryo to form, starting with the spine and head.
- The formation of the placenta: The placenta, which is the main source of nourishment for the embryo, is developed by about the third month. The embryo is connected with the placenta by the umbilical cord — a thick string of skin containing 2 arteries and a vein — through which all nourishment, oxygen, as well as waste products, pass. (Point to placenta and development of umbilical cord in Picture 16).
- Miscarriage: A defective embryo is expelled by our bodies, most often during the first 3 months. This is called a miscarriage. It is important that the uterus is cleaned out after a miscarriage as otherwise, an infection may start. If you have a miscarriage, you should go to a clinic immediately.

The food we need and what to avoid — Pictures 17-19

Discussion points:

- Your body needs enough to grow a healthy baby. You also need plenty of fluids.
- Food groups (Picture 17): To grow a healthy baby, we need to eat a mixed diet of cereals (grains, rice, wheat, corn), fruits/vegetables (leafy green vegetables and potatoes, carrots, yams); and proteins (beans, meat, fish).
- What to avoid: What we eat and drink, and put into our bodies is passed on to the developing embryo and fetus through the placenta, and affects the baby. Therefore, smoking is not only bad for you but it is a hazard for the developing baby. Alcohol may damage the unborn baby.
- Drugs: If you have to take drugs of any kind on doctor's orders, tell the doctor as soon as you are pregnant; perhaps your prescription should be changed. Drugs and medicines may affect the growth and development of the embryo and fetus, and the health of your child after birth.
- Discuss don'ts in more detail, depending on the country/environment/group, with whom you work.

Picture 19: To go with the pictures you put here, talk about available healthy foodstuffs in your area and their costs. This provides the opportunity for a general discussion on nutrition in relation to local foods and eating habits. Your presentation should be carefully researched, about food practices of the target group and based on locally available foods. Discuss recipes of familiar foods and/or how to change them to make a more nourishing meal.

Development of pregnancy — Pictures 20-22

Discussion points:

- The first 6 months (Picture 20, top row): The body shows few visible signs of pregnancy. Most of the changes take place on the inside. (Refer to discussion of Pictures 15/16 "Changes")
- The last 3 months (Picture 20, bottom row): The abdomen expands a great deal as the fetus grows rapidly inside the uterus.
- Enlargement of breasts: The nipples enlarge and the area around them gets darker early in pregnancy. The breasts enlarge as the milk glands grow and get ready for milk production.
- Movement of the fetus: After about 20 weeks we begin to feel the fetus move – at first, very slightly. Later, the movements get stronger. We can feel the fetus "kick" inside the amniotic sac, where it can move about freely in the amniotic fluid.
- Point out changes in appearance of embryo, fetus, umbilical cord, growth of breasts, etc. Show how in the last figure of Picture 20 (bottom right) the baby has "dropped".

Just before birth and beginning of labor — Pictures 23, 24

Discussion points:

- Fetus fully developed: During the last month, the fetus is fully developed and puts on more weight and a layer of fat. Picture 23: show the umbilical cord, placenta, position of fetus, etc.
- Cervix closed: The opening of the uterus towards the vagina is still completely closed. The head of the fetus is in the usual birth position (pointing down) as in 96% of deliveries.
- Baby moves into position: Note in Picture 24 the changes in the position of the baby in the figures on the left. In the second picture the baby has "dropped". Point to the change in the cervix and the change in the appearance of the abdomen.
- Labor: The contractions of the uterus to push the baby out are called "labor". The contractions, which we cannot control, start when the baby is ready to be born. Picture 24 (upper right figure), shows how the uterus pushes down during a contraction.
- First stage of labor: the contractions of the uterus open the cervix to the birth canal (vagina) to let the baby out.
- Timing of contractions: At first, the contractions are about half an hour apart and gradually become more frequent. When they are about 2 minutes apart you will soon be ready to deliver. Labor with a first baby may take from several hours to more than a day; subsequent babies may be born much quicker.
- The contractions of the uterus to open the cervix cause labor pains. Discuss here breathing techniques, relaxation, walking around during labor. Tension and fear increase pain. Support and encouragement from your husband/partner, mother, or friends is important.
- Prevention of pain: What drugs against pain are safe for mother and baby? Discuss what drugs are available in your country/area, how they are taken, and what they do. Other methods to prevent pain (see above).
- Preparation for childbirth: Discuss what preparations are needed in your area — home birth, hospital birth, where/how to find midwife/doctor, birth attendant; family support, etc.

The birth process — Pictures 25, 26

Discussion points:

- The birth position: the position shows a woman with her back propped up, which lets her push the baby down; thus the weight of the baby helps to push it out.
- The first stage of labor: In the upper row of Picture 25, the cervix, the door to the uterus, is opening up. The contractions, which are very painful, push the head of the baby against the cervix to dilate it or open it up. Breathing deeply and slowly helps to control the pain.
- The bag of waters breaks and the fluid which has surrounded the baby comes out. This can happen before or after contractions begin. This is different with each delivery.
- The second stage of labor: In the lower row of figures of Picture 25, the cervix is open and the baby is pushed through the birth canal. During this second stage of labor, you can help by pushing with each contraction to make the baby come out.
- Crowning: (Picture 26, top row). Crowning means the baby's head starts to come out. The skinfolds around the opening of the vagina are soft and elastic, to let the head through. The baby's head turns through the birth canal, which makes it easier to come out. It is better not to push too hard at this last stage of labor so that the skin around the opening does not tear.
- Emergence of the head: if the skin is not sufficiently elastic, or the baby's head is too large, the skin surrounding the vaginal opening may tear. To prevent tearing, an "episiotomy" may be made; that is, a cut into the skin surrounding the opening. In most cases, if you wait, the skin will stretch and the head will come out with no damage to the mother or baby.

Birth positions and birth — Pictures 27, 28

Discussion points:

- Birth Positions: In different parts of the world, women give birth in different ways and positions. Picture 27 shows some positions women use to make birth easier. Birth positions vary with local customs and traditions. Some birth traditions may be useful; others may be damaging. Local traditions relating to birth should be carefully reviewed before teaching something different or new.
- What is the best position? The best position is the one that is most comfortable for you. Between contractions, you can walk around, eat or drink, and rest. Make yourself comfortable in whatever way you think best for you. Lying flat on your back, with your knees up and your legs held in stirrups, (the Lithotomy position) which used to be common in many hospitals, makes it harder to give birth because the baby has to be pushed up. The position in most of the pictures is half-sitting, with the back supported: this way the weight of the baby helps with the delivery. In this position, the baby is pushed down.
- Childbirth needs support: Birth is hard work for the mother, who needs support, encouragement and caring from those close to her: her husband/partner, and family. It is a long process that needs patience and skilled help, and in case of an emergency, professional or hospital back-up.
- Birth (Picture 28): The baby's head is usually born first. Most of the time, a baby begins to cry at once, as soon as its lungs fill with air. If the baby's nose and mouth are blocked with mucus, this should be removed at once. If the baby doesn't breathe, mouth-to-mouth respiration must be given immediately.
- The baby's head is still soft and sometimes may be out of shape from being pushed through the birth canal. The head will recover its normal shape in a few days.
- The umbilical cord is still attached to the placenta (afterbirth), inside the uterus, and the baby may be wet and covered with a white substance called vernix. The baby should be handed to the mother to hold at once, or placed on her abdomen, to establish the first bonds of love and care.

Immediate newborn care and afterbirth — Pictures 29, 30

Discussion points:

- The newborn is breathing after the mucus has been cleaned from its mouth and nose; the baby is handed to the mother to hold. Within the first hour of life, the baby should eat at her breast.
- Cutting of cord: After the cord, still attached to the placenta, stops pulsating, it is tied in 2 places (one close to the baby). Then the cord is cut between the ties with sterile scissors or a sterile razor blade.
- The stump of the cord will fall off in a few days. It should be kept dry and clean; nothing should be put on the stump. The drier it is, the sooner it will fall off.
- Breastfeeding: The baby is usually alert after the birth, and should breastfeed within the first hour of life. The first milk is called colostrum. It is loaded with antibodies to protect the baby against disease, and it provides nourishment. Nursing stimulates the breasts so that they produce more milk. The baby needs only breast milk, no other fluids or solids, for the first 6 months of life.
- Afterbirth (Placenta): (Picture 30). A short time after the baby has been born, the afterbirth is expelled by a few more contractions from the uterus. The belly may be gently massaged so the placenta is detached from the uterus. Do not pull on the cord. If the placenta does not come out after half an hour, get help from a hospital or maternity clinic.
- Bleeding: Some loss of blood by the mother is normal, quite aside from the placenta. If bleeding is strong or continues after delivery, this can be dangerous and help in a hospital should be sought. Normal bleeding (as during menstruation) continues for several weeks.
- Weight and size of the baby: A baby that weighs less than 5 lb (2 kg) needs special attention and care. Average size and weight of a baby is different with different population groups. The baby's size and weight also is influenced by the size of the parents, the nourishment/health of mother, the length of pregnancy, etc.

Breastfeeding — Pictures 31, 32

Discussion points:

- Breastfeeding: the mother should breastfeed her baby within the first hour of life. The first milk, colostrum, prevents infections and is an important form of nourishment for the baby. When the baby nurses, this stimulates more milk production. Sometimes the mother feels cramping with breastfeeding at first, especially if this is not her first baby. This is healthy – it means the breastfeeding is helping the uterus contract and go back to its usual size.
- Breastfeeding positions: (Picture 31). There are many different positions to nurse a baby; you and your baby should be comfortable and nursing should not hurt. The baby should open the mouth widely and take in a large part of the breast.
- Risks to not breastfeeding: Human milk protects the baby against many sicknesses and gives the baby the best chance of survival. Artificial milks and animal milks have health risks for the baby. The most nutritionally complete alternative is infant formula, but if clean water, sterilization, and refrigeration are not available, it is not a safe alternative.
- Food for a breastfeeding mother: Your own body needs a balanced diet; that is, a variety of foods (Picture 32).
- Review discussion of Pictures 17, 18, and 19 "The Food We Need", "What to Avoid", and "Familiar Foods". The same nutrition is needed for a nursing mother as during pregnancy. What a mother eats/drinks is passed on to the baby through her milk.

- Feeding the baby: The baby needs nothing except your milk for the first 6 months of life. At 6 months you can start to add solid foods such as cereals, mashed fruit (such as bananas, applesauce, etc), cooked and mashed vegetables, and whatever soft foods you eat yourself. You also can buy ready-made baby foods in many stores.

Unusual positions of the baby and multiple births — Picture 33

Discussion points:

- Unusual positions: The 3 women on the left are carrying their babies in unusual positions. It is possible sometimes (by a trained midwife or doctor) to turn the baby around before birth. Being born feet first is called a "breech" birth (second figure from left). Some providers with a lot of experience can help breech babies to be born without surgery, but in most nations with modern hospitals, breech births are delivered under anesthesia in hospital by cesarean section; that means, cutting open the mother's abdomen and uterus, and taking the baby out. The most difficult position is transverse (third figure from left): a Cesarean section will need to be done. At the end of the pregnancy, if a woman's baby is in an unusual position, she should go to a maternity hospital because the delivery may be difficult and dangerous for her and for the baby.
- Twins and multiple births: There are 2 kinds of twins: identical twins (formed from one egg cell) who share a placenta, are the same sex, and look almost exactly alike. Twins from 2 egg cells have their own placenta, and may be of different sex and different appearance.

  Sometimes even more babies than 2 grow at one time: triplets (3 babies) or quadruplets (4 babies) are much more rarely born, and often are so small that they are unable to survive without specialized care in an intensive care unit.
- How do you know if you will have twins? The large size of the abdomen may show you carry more than one baby. More than one heart beat can be heard towards the end of pregnancy if you are examined by a midwife or doctor. Sometimes twins run in families – if you have lots of twins in your family, you may be more likely to have twins, but this is not always true. You should go to a hospital for delivery if you think you carry more than one child.

Family planning and contraception — Picture 34

Discussion points:

- Explain all contraceptives shown. Point to each picture and outline how the different contraceptives are used.
- Indicate which contraceptives are available locally and where.
- Explain birth spacing / family planning. The body needs rest after delivery. Many pregnancies in quick succession deplete a mother's strength and may result in unhealthy, damaged or stillborn babies.
- Call on local family planning organization to give a presentation on locally used family planning methods and show contraceptives and their use. Or, get family planning information/teaching materials/contraceptives from local family planning organization to demonstrate.

THE CHILDBIRTH PICTURE BOOK

GLOSSARY

A

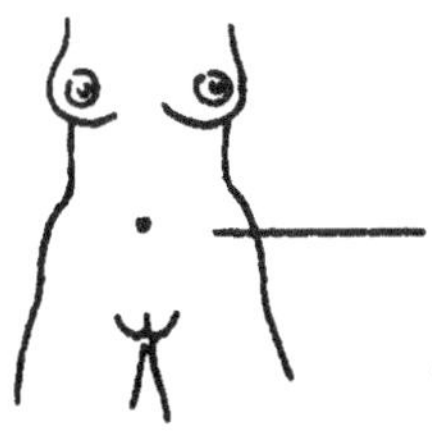

Abdomen and pelvis
The area between the breasts and the legs, containing the genital organs.

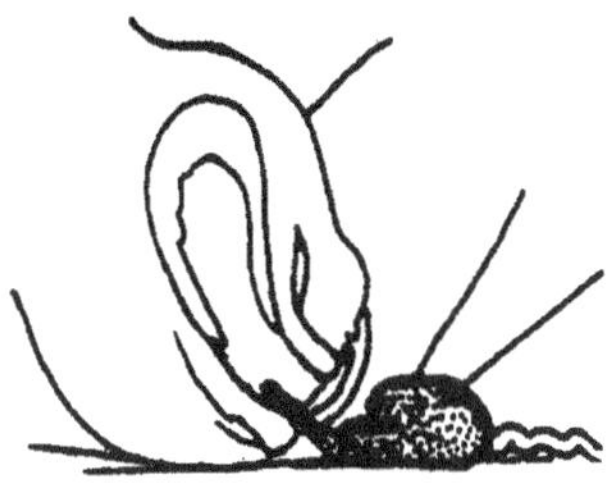

Afterbirth
The expulsion of the placenta and the contents of the uterus after the baby has been delivered.

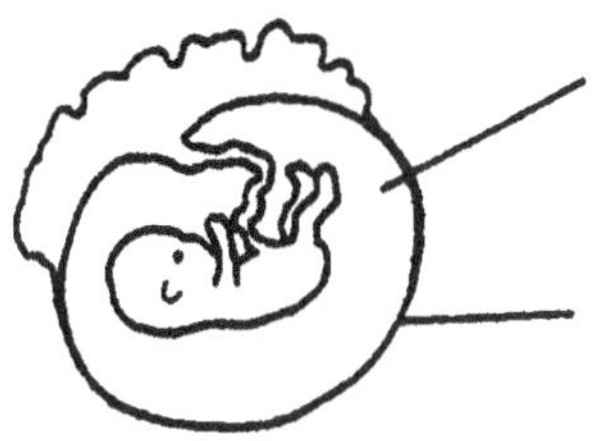

Amniotic fluid
The liquid which surrounds the baby inside the amniotic sac.

Amniotic sac
The sac inside of which the embryo/fetus grows surrounded by fluid. It develops inside the uterus from the cover of the egg cell.

B

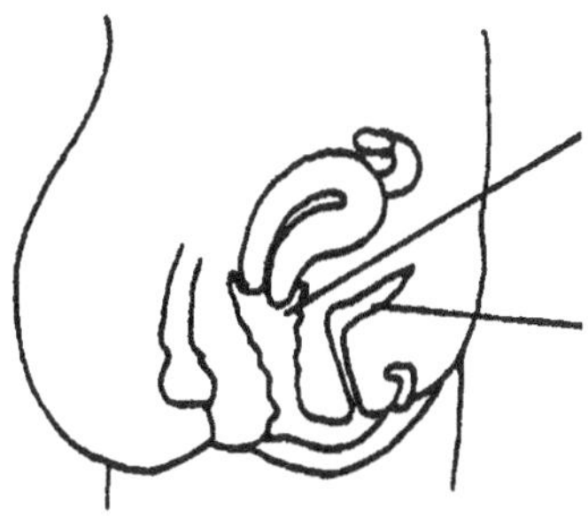

Birth canal or vagina
The canal between the uterus and the outside, through which the baby must be pushed.

Bladder
A hollow sac where urine is stored, inside the abdomen.

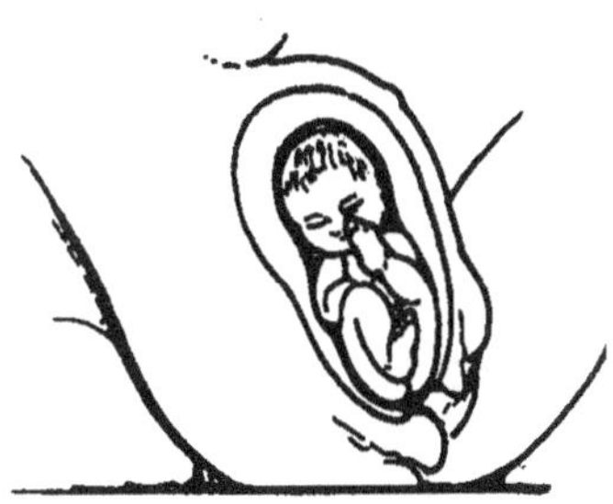

Breech birth
The birth of a baby that is born feet first, or head last. Needs special assistance.

C

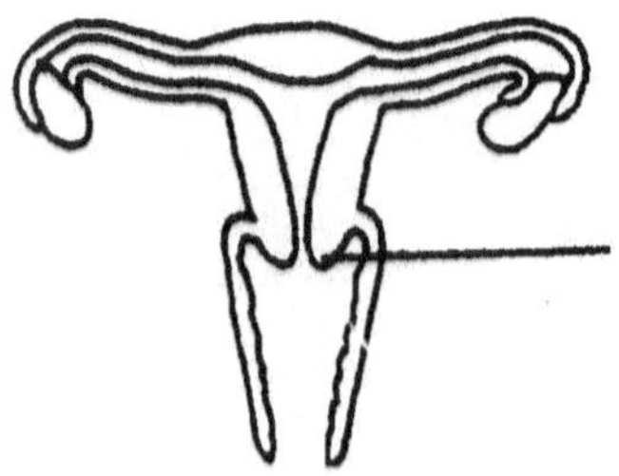

Cervix
The small opening of the uterus (womb) to the vagina/birth canal.

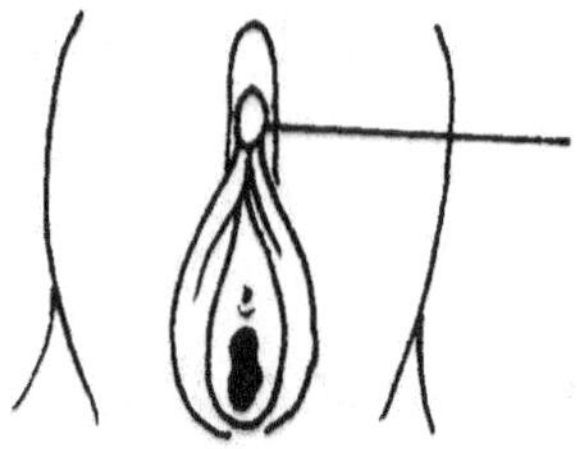

Clitoris
The most sensitive organ of the female body, located in front of the vaginal opening. The female sexual nerve center, similar to the penis in males.

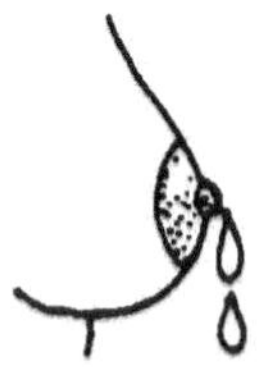

Colostrum
The first milk. It may be clear or yellow, or any color in between. It is packed with antibodies and nutrients and very important for the health of the baby.

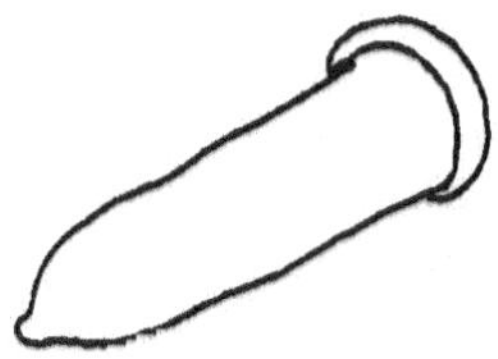

Condom or sheath
A thin rubber or latex cover worn over the penis to prevent sperm cells from entering the vagina and uterus during intercourse, and to prevent passing infections such as HIV and other STIs.

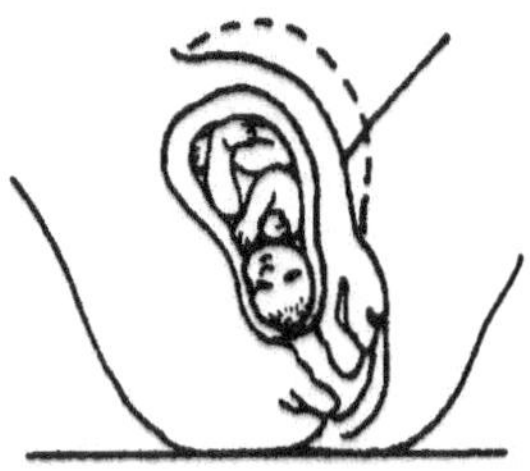

Contractions of the uterus
Pains (or cramps) in regular intervals that begin the birth process. Contractions of the uterus usually start about a half-hour apart. When they are 2 minutes apart, the delivery is about to begin.

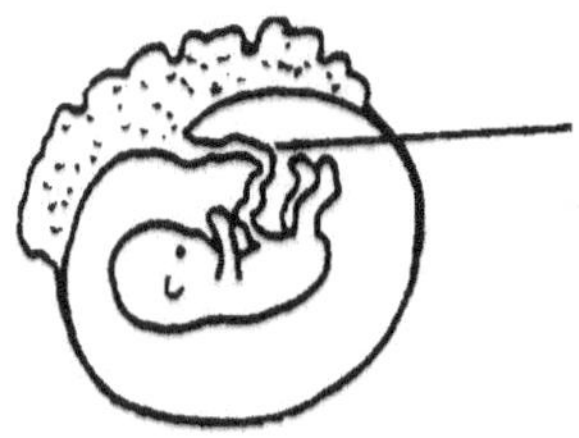

Cord (umbilical)
A tube of skin through which all nourishment and waste products flow from the placenta to the fetus, and back. The "lifeline" of the fetus.

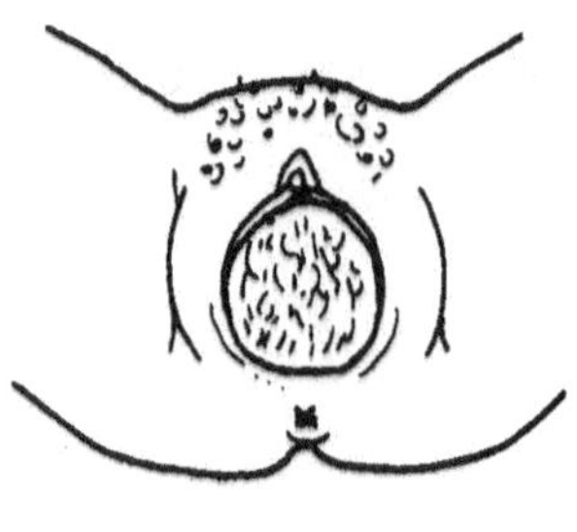

Crowning
The stretching of the skin of the vaginal opening, around the baby's head, just before the head comes out.

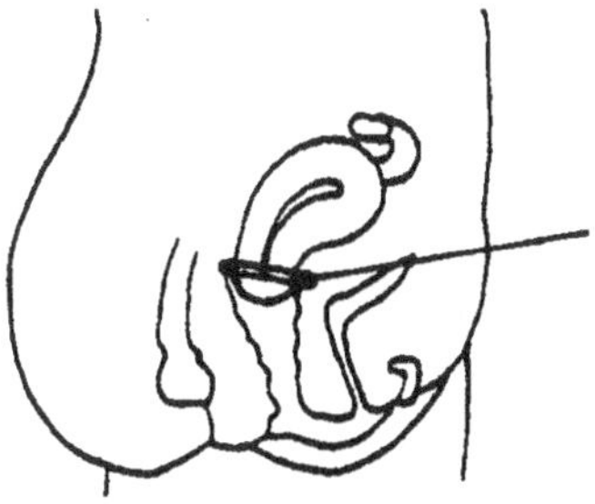

D

Diaphragm

A plastic cap that closes the opening of the uterus (cervix) and prevents pregnancy.

E

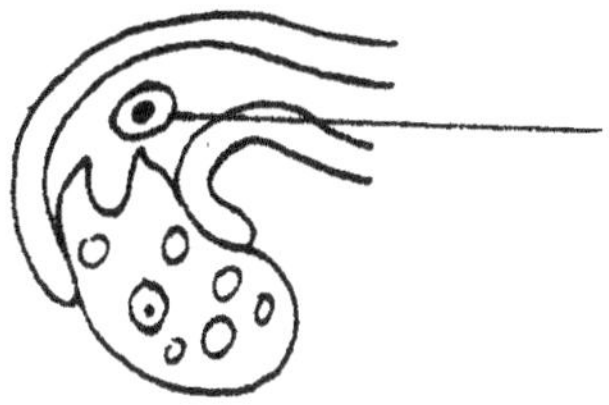

Egg cell or ovum

The largest cell of our bodies, capable of reproducing itself after it is fertilized by a sperm cell.

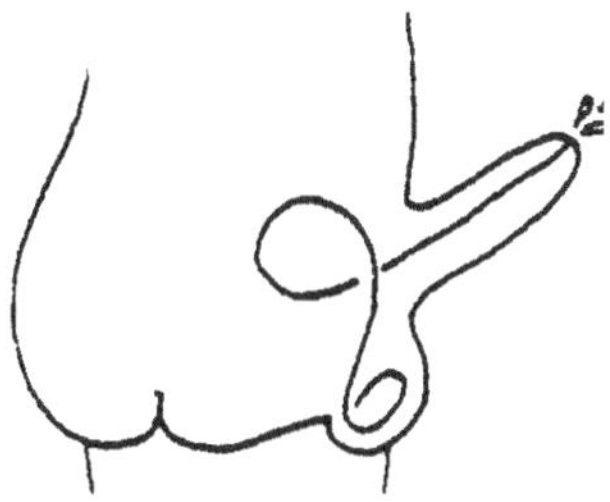

Ejaculation

The ejection (expulsion) of the male sperm cells, contained in a liquid called semen, from the penis.

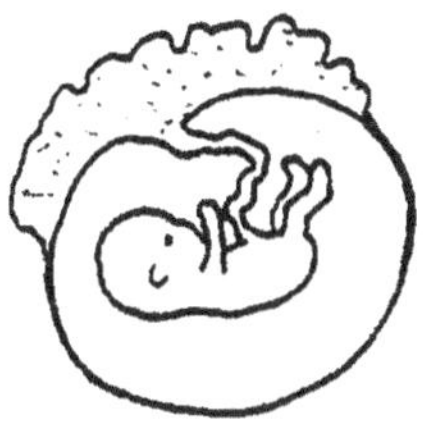

Embryo

The early stages in the development of any organism. In human anatomy the term is applied to the developing ovum in the first 2 months, or until it shows any human characteristics.

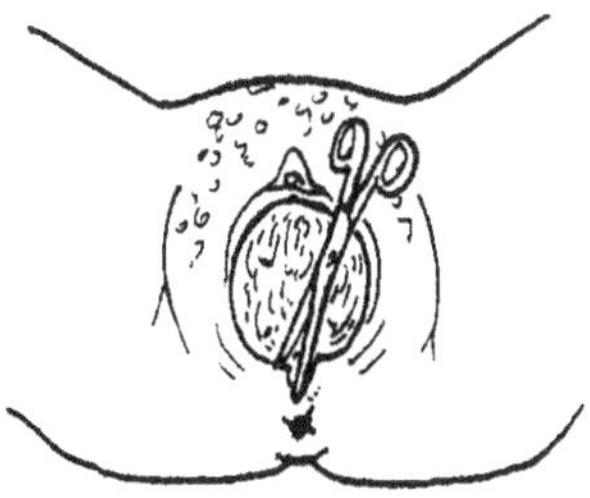

Episiotomy

An incision that is made in the perineum, the skin around the opening of the vagina, to let the baby's head out, when the opening cannot stretch enough.

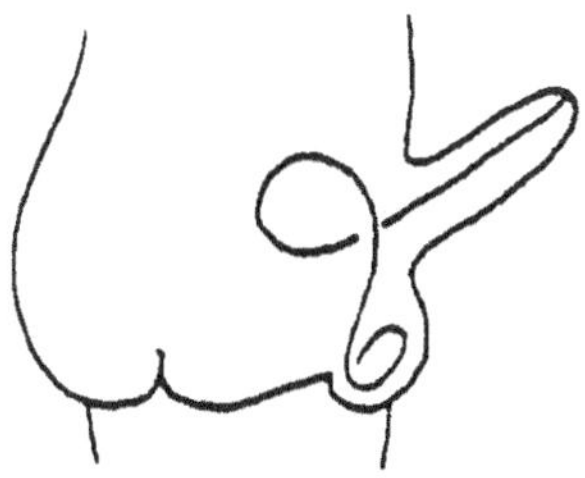

Erection

The enlarged, rigid penis, standing out from the body. Erection is due to sexual excitement.

F

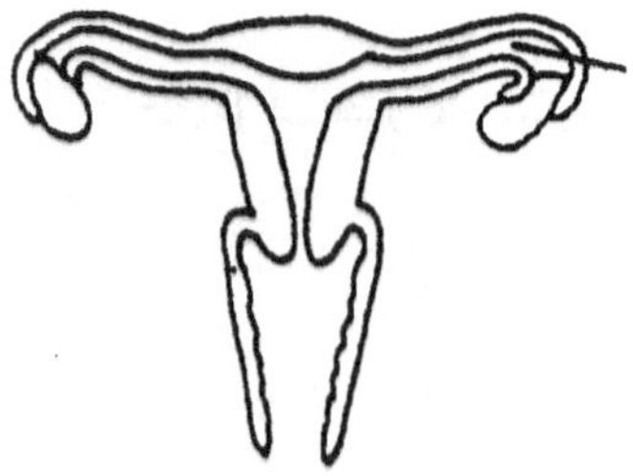

Fallopian tube

A hollow passageway that connects the uterus with the ovary, the container of egg cells. We have 2 Fallopian tubes, through which a ripe egg cell moves from one ovary to the uterus, once a month.

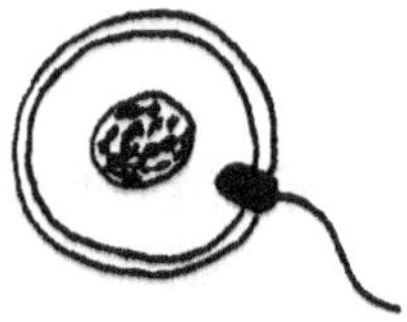

Fertilization

Takes place when a male sperm cell penetrates a ripe egg cell and combines with it. This is also called "impregnation".

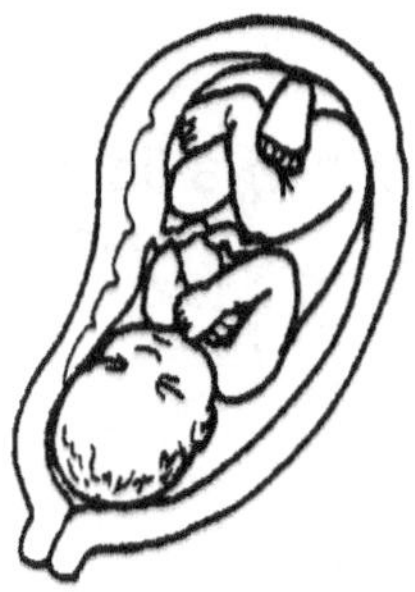

Fetus

An unborn baby inside the uterus. This term is usually used with the third month of pregnancy.

G

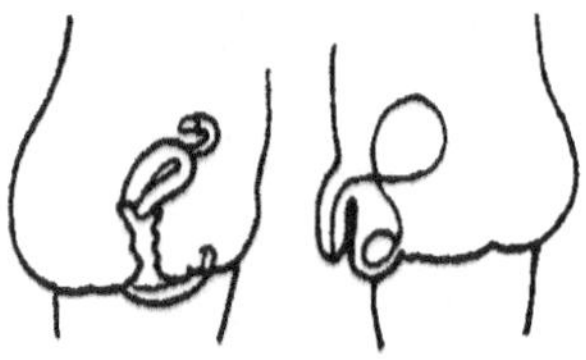

Genital organs

The female and male organs directly involved with reproduction.

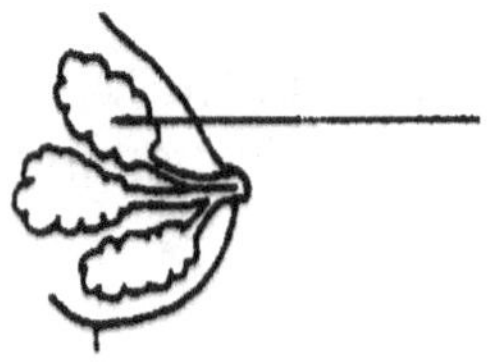

Gland

An organ capable of producing a substance: the milk glands in the breasts produce milk.

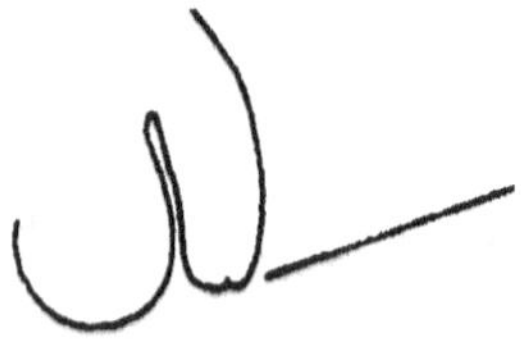

Glans

The round tip of the penis which is very sensitive and has many nerve endings, similar to the clitoris in females.

I

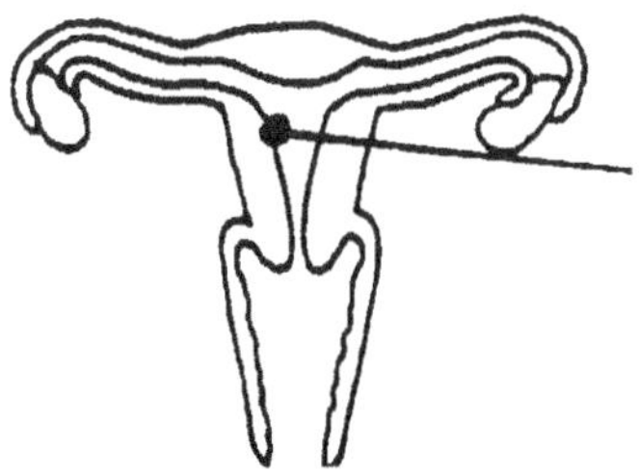

Implantation
The attachment of the fertilized egg cell to the lining of the uterus.

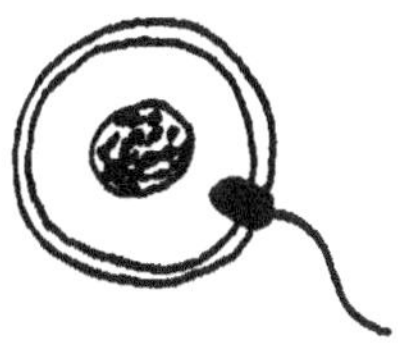

Impregnation or fertilization
To make pregnant or to fertilize a ripe egg cell by combination with a sperm cell.

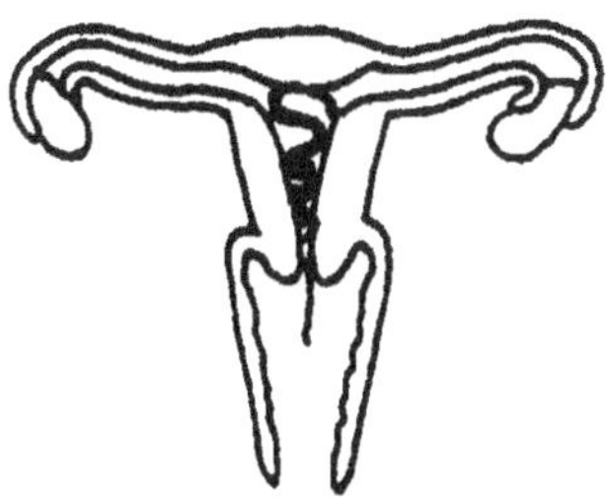

IUD/Intrauterine device
A plastic coil or device inserted in the uterus, which prevents pregnancy.

L

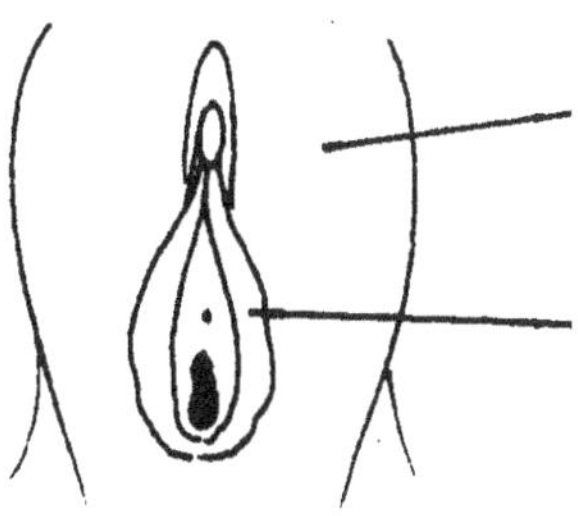

Labia majora ('big lips')
Outer skinfolds covering the entrance to the vagina and urinary opening.

Labia minora ('small lips')
Inner skinfolds covering the entrance to the vagina and urinary opening

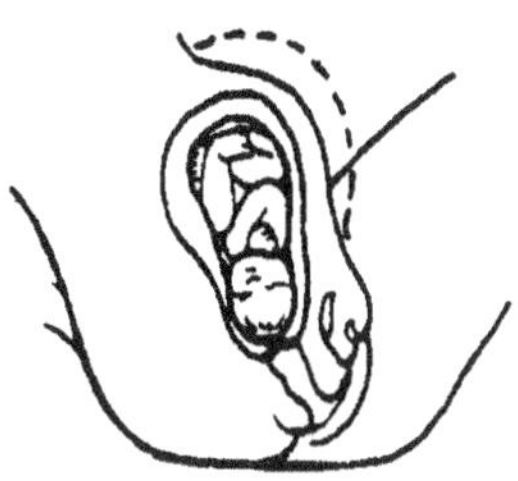

Labor
The act of giving birth. The regular contractions (cramps) of the uterus, to expel the baby. (See Contractions).

M

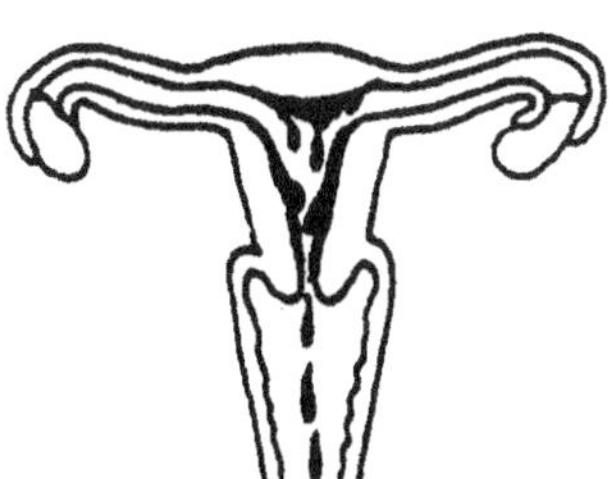

Menstruation
The monthly elimination of the blood-filled lining of the uterus (womb), which takes about 45 days.

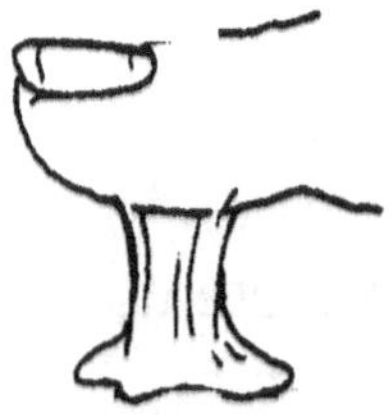

Mucus

A sticky substance made by mucus glands that sometimes clogs the newborn baby's nose and mouth, and should be removed.

O

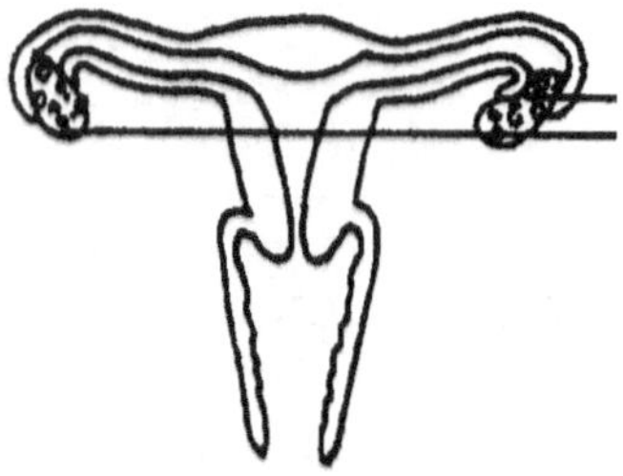

Ovary

A pair of organs or glands inside the abdomen, containing the egg cells. After puberty, one egg cell each month ripens and is released from the ovary.

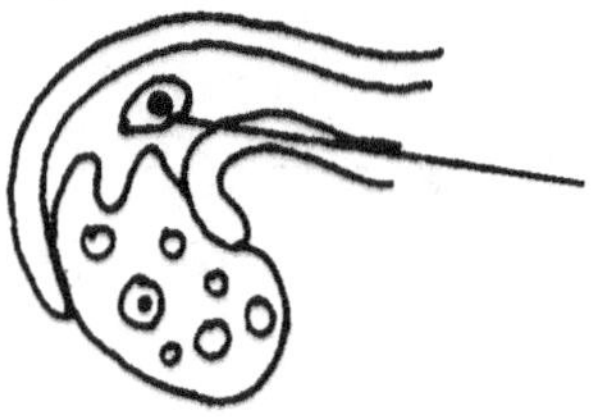

Ovulation

The release of a ripe egg cell from the ovary (about once a month).

Ovum

An egg cell — the largest cell of our body. Capable of reproduction, when fertilized.

P

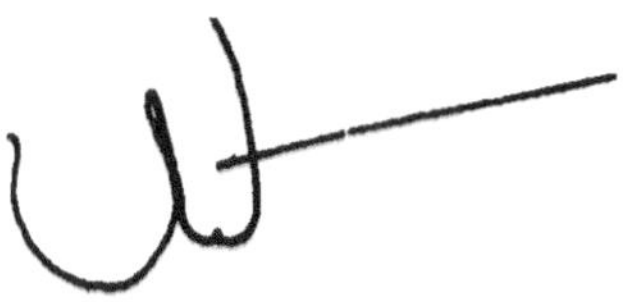

Penis

A tube-shaped male organ that is used for elimination of urine and which ejaculates (releases) sperm cells after sexual excitement.

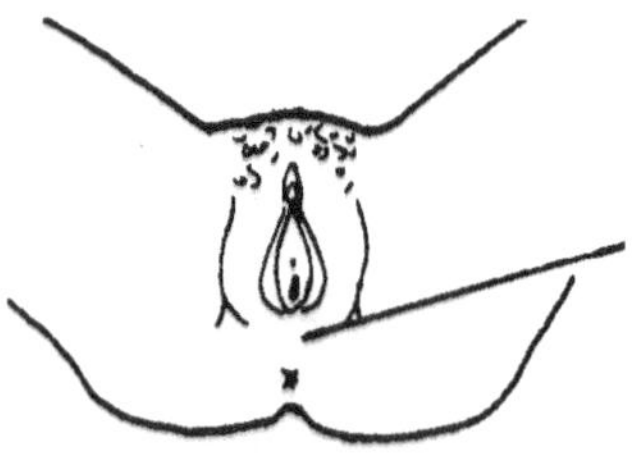

Perineum

The area of skin and muscles between the opening of the vagina and the anus.

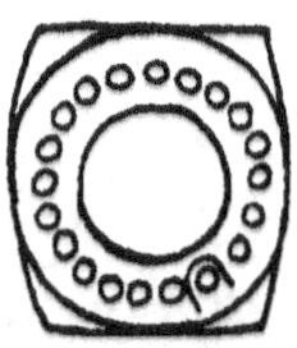

The "Pill"

A pill taken regularly to prevent pregnancy.

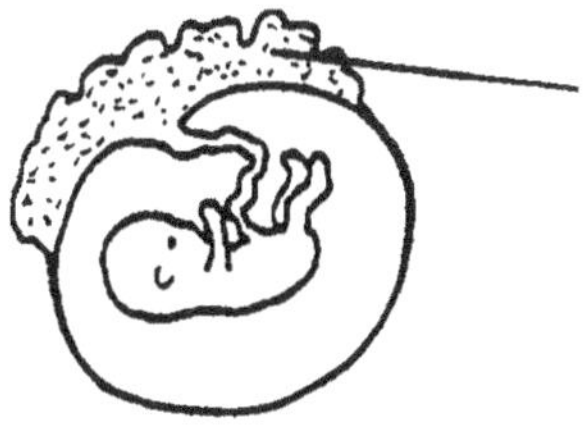

Placenta

A special organ formed by about the third month of pregnancy. Through the placenta, our body supplies the fetus with nourishment and gets rid of waste products.

S

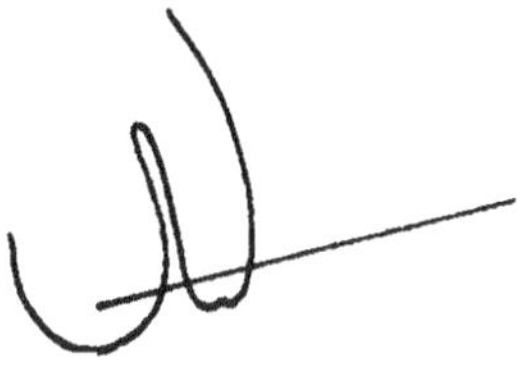

Scrotum

The protective sac that contains the 2 testicles of a man. (See Testicles).

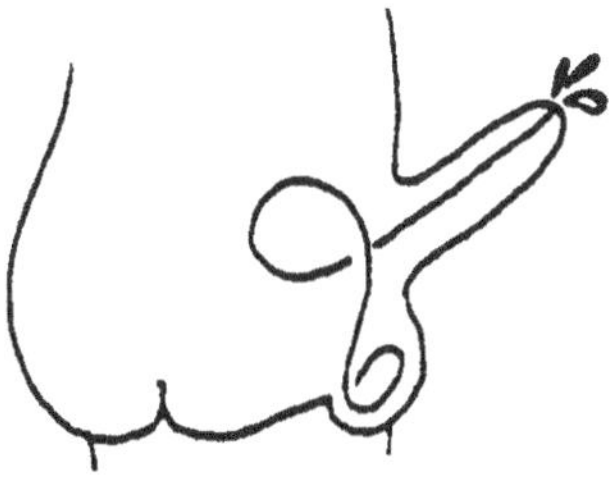

Semen

A milky liquid full of sperm cells, coming out of the penis during ejaculation (See Ejaculation).

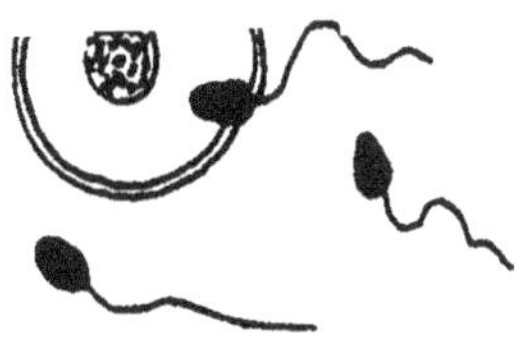

Sperm cell

The male seed produced inside the testicles, which is needed to fertilize an egg. It consists of a head or nucleus and a tail.

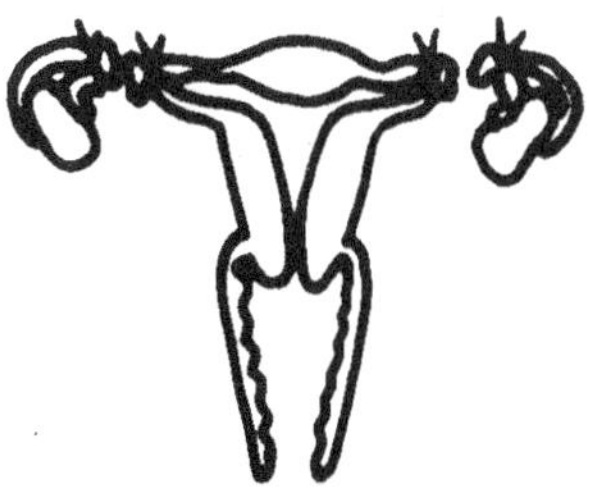

Sterilization: female

Tubal ligation: cutting of the Fallopian tubes so that egg cells cannot enter the uterus and the woman can not become pregnant again.

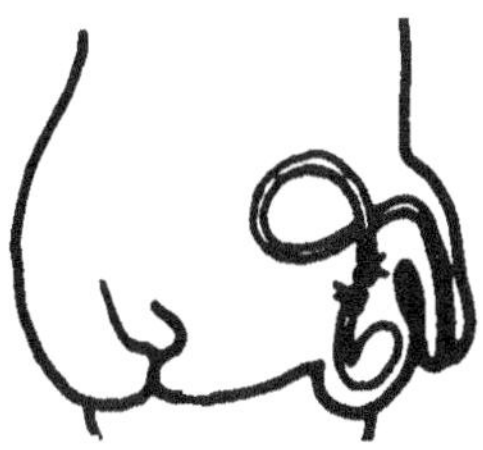

Sterilization: male

Vasectomy: cutting of the vas deferens, through which sperm cells reach the penis, so that they are not ejaculated.

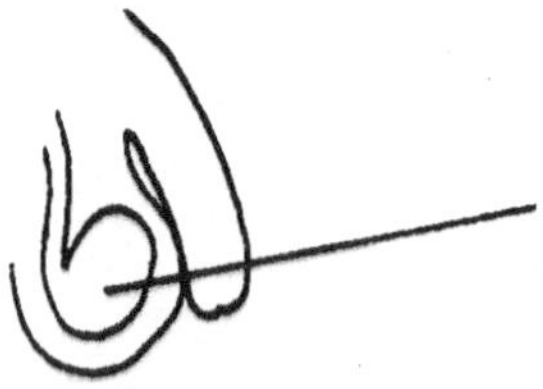

T

Testicles

The 2 male glands which produce sperm cells. They are inside the protective sac of the scrotum.

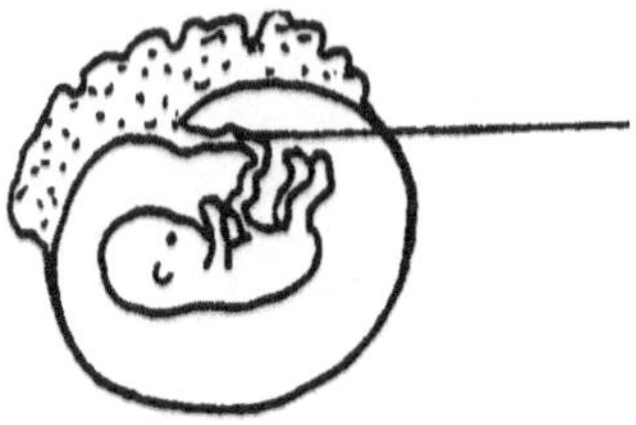

U

Umbilical cord

A tube of skin through which all nourishment and waste products flow from the placenta to the fetus and back. The "life line" of the fetus. (See Cord).

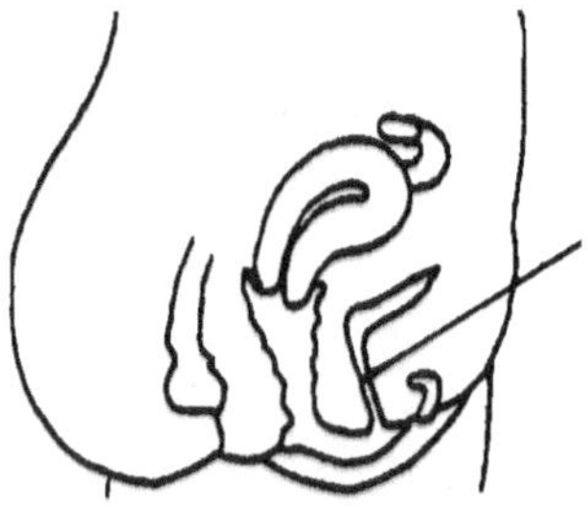

Urethra

The duct to the bladder through which urine is eliminated — located between vaginal opening and clitoris.

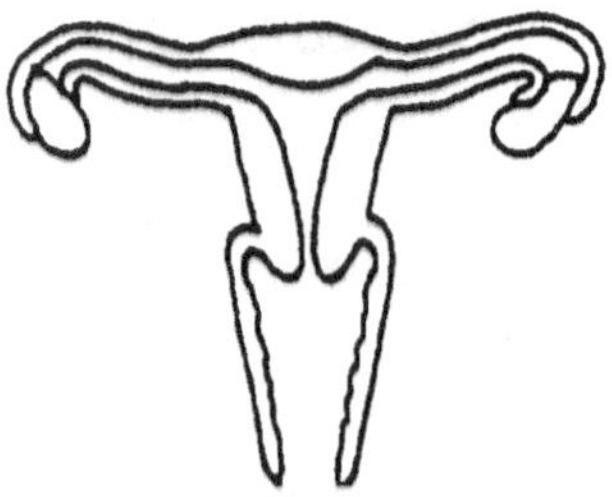

Urethral meatus (opening of urethra)

Opening of duct to bladder through which urine is eliminated.

Uterus or womb

Oblong, pear-shaped, hollow muscle. Inside the uterus, the embryo/fetus develops until it is ready to be born.

V

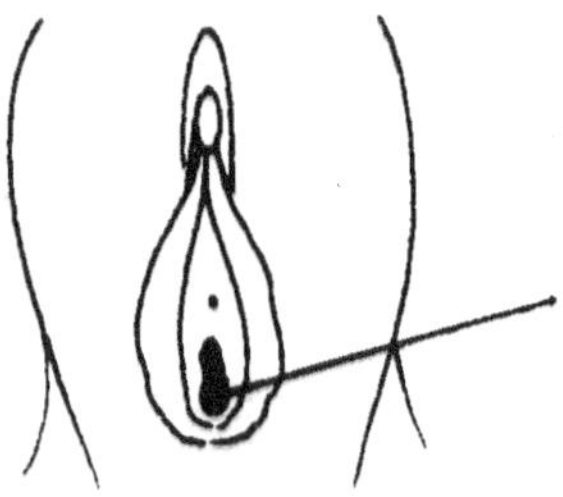

Vagina

Oblong, tube-shaped, hollow organ leading to uterus (womb).

Vaginal opening

Opening of vagina located between anus and urethral opening.

Vulva

The exterior genital organs of a woman.

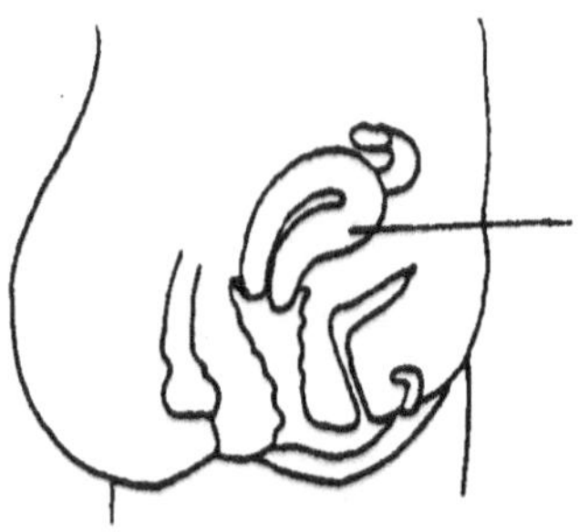

W

Womb

A hollow, oblong muscle that contains the baby during its development (See Uterus).

THE CHILDBIRTH PICTURE BOOK

Acknowledgements

We would like to express our thanks to Dr. Gordon Wallace, a longtime friend of Fran Hosken's, and to the Wallace Global Fund for their ongoing financial support of this program.

We would also like to thank Kathy Dillon for her work and long term support of Fran's projects.

Fran also paid tribute to the following people for their assistance: Mary Lee Garrant, LPN; Susan C. Marchessault, Janet Isaacs Ashford, Judith Luce, Trudy Cox, Linda Collins, the Boston Women's Health Book Collective, and to African and Asian midwives Khin Mu Aye, Temperance Lolaka, Rosalyn Owino, and Marie Toure Ngom.

Translations and adaptations

The Childbirth Picture Book is available from Hesperian in Arabic, English, French Somali, and Spanish. The CPB has been adapted and printed in India by CHETNA in Hindi, Gujarati, Telugu and Bengali, printed in Ethiopia, and serialized in Bangladesh and Haiti. The Marimed Foundation sponsored a translation into Marshallese.

Hesperian welcomes initiatives to translate and adapt these teaching materials. They are copyrighted to prevent commercial exploitation: the use of the copyright is made readily available to organizations interested in reprinting for nonprofit educational use. Please contact Hesperian for further information.